Current Practice in
Health Sciences Librarianship

Alison Bunting
Editor-in-Chief

Volume 4
Collection Development and Assessment
in Health Sciences Libraries

by
Daniel T. Richards
and
Dottie Eakin

Medical Library Association
and
The Scarecrow Press, Inc.
Lanham, Md., & London

SCARECROW PRESS, INC.

Published in the United States of America
by Scarecrow Press, Inc.
4720 Boston Way
Lanham, Maryland 20706

4 Pleydell Gardens, Folkestone
Kent CT20 2DN, England

British Cataloguing-in-Publication Information Available

Library of Congress Cataloging-in-Publication Data

Richards, Daniel T.
    Collection development and assessment in health sciences libraries
  / by Daniel T. Richards and Dottie Eakin.
        p.   cm. — (Current practice in health sciences librarianship ; v. 4)
    Includes bibliographical references and index.
    ISBN 0-8108-3201-1 (alk. paper)
      1. Medical libraries—Collection development—United States.
    I. Eakin, Dottie. II. Title. III. Series.
    Z675.M4R53   1996
    026.61—dc20   96-31662

ISBN 0-8108-3201-1 (cloth: alk. paper)

Printed in the United States of America

        The paper used in this publication meets the minimum requirements of
American National Standard for Information Sciences—Permanence of Paper for
Printed Library Materials, ANSI Z39.48-1984.

This book is dedicated to

LOUISE DARLING

for her friendship,
expert guidance,
counsel,
and wisdom
which she has provided in abundance over the years
and
which have shaped our careers in medical librarianship.

Dan Richards, 1945-1995

Dan Richards, whose idea it was to write this book, left us unexpectedly as it was in its final pre-publication stages. Our last interactions were the hours huddling together over the book galleys in the Washington Hilton. Even the task of finding the perfect turn of phrase and correcting each other's grammar was enjoyable, as all work with Dan was fun.

No one was more intensely intertwined with collection development in health sciences libraries than Dan. He was a founder of the collection development section of the Medical Library Association. He developed and taught a popular continuing education course in assessment of health sciences library collections. He wrote articles and book chapters on collection development topics and co-compiled a published set of sample collection policies. He guided the revision of the National Library of Medicine's collection policy. It was his ideas and actions that resulted in two collection development symposia. He served as an advisor to Wiley Publishing and *Doody's Health Sciences Book Review Journal.*

It was Dan's idea to honor our mutual teacher and mentor, Louise Darling, by establishing the Louise Darling Medal for Distinguished Achievement in Collection Development in the Health Sciences and assuring that it was endowed. He was the proud recipient of the second medal awarded. As a member of the MLA Books Panel, Dan was a strong supporter of the recommendation that the name of this series' predecessor, the *Handbook of Medical Library Practice*, be updated to *Current Practice in Health Sciences Librarianship.*

Dan's long experience, his great knowledge, and his critical thinking shine throughout the pages of this book, enlightening the reader. There will be no replacing either his contributions or the wonderful, bigger-than-life, person he was.

Dottie Eakin
Alison Bunting

Collection Development and Assessment in Health Sciences Libraries

Contents

Preface

Current Practice in Health Sciences Librarianship (CPHSL) continues the publication principles established by its predecessor, the *Handbook of Medical Library Practice*, to serve as: a general introduction to the field of health sciences librarianship for graduate students; a source of basic information and references to the literature for the Medical Library Association's (MLA) professional development and recognition program; a reference work for health sciences librarians and other information specialists, providing basic information in areas peripheral to their own expertise; and a means of documenting the state of practice of health sciences librarianship at a particular point in time.

The decision to change the title of this venerable MLA publication is best explained by a review of the *Handbook*'s publication history. The appearance in 1942 of the first edition of the *Handbook*, published by the American Library Association, fulfilled a long-standing goal of the MLA. As editor Janet Doe noted,

> The demand [for a Handbook] has grown keener with the passage of time, undoubtedly because of the recent rapid increase in the number of medical libraries, for half of the 315 now existing in this country have originated since 1910. To staff these libraries, workers have been enticed or commandeered from general and special libraries, from library schools, from the clerical staff of hospitals or medical schools, and from doctors' offices [1].

The second edition of the *Handbook* (1956), edited by Janet Doe and Mary Louise Marshall [2], updated the one-volume first edition, retaining, whenever possible, the original chapter authors. The preface to this volume included an apology for publication delays and noted that some of the information in the volume was written three or more years prior to publication.

Fourteen years elapsed before the third edition, the first one published by MLA, appeared in 1970. Editors Gertrude L. Annan and Jacqueline W. Felter took an entirely different approach: "The chapters are written by a new cadre of authors and differ from those of the earlier edition in substance and emphasis"[3]. Despite the expansion of the scope and coverage, the one volume format was retained. Four consultants from different types of health sciences libraries ensured that the content took into account library practice in these settings. Publication delays continued to be a problem and were

> ...of grave concern to the editors who regret that some chapters were written several years before the volume went to press. With so many involved in the preparation of the work, unforeseen emergencies arose which prevented its production in the period scheduled [4].

Louise Darling, David Bishop, and Lois Ann Colaianni edited the fourth edition, published between 1982 and 1988. This edition included a "...shift in terminology from medical to health science libraries...in it-self...indicative of the new complexity, the highly interdisciplinary nature of the fields served by these libraries"[5]. However, the title of the Handbook was not changed "...because of the risk of obscuring the continuity of editions"[6]. A three-volume format was chosen to: "...accommodate material on new developments, lessen the delays inherent in a multiple-author work, and facilitate later revision..."[7]. This new approach did not, however, prevent publication delays

> ...even with a smaller number of authors per volume, the consid-erable time difference in submission of chapters has meant that the problem of keeping material within the volume on the same level of currency, though reduced, has not been solved [8].

And, "...the sequential publication has resulted in problems of uneven currency in the completed work..."[9]. "A more satisfactory method for revising the Handbook in the future is now under study, as the rapid pace of change in the information field obviously requires a new approach"[10].

In 1989, the MLA Books Panel recommended that the Handbook be continued with the same general scope and content as the fourth edition, but that the three volumes be further divided into a series of smaller monographs, each dealing with a single subject and each with its own volume editor. An editor-in-chief, assisted by an Advisory Committee, was appointed to coordinate the publication. The Advisory Committee deter-mined that health sciences librarianship is changing so rapidly that the profession will be better served by publication of a series, and that the series required a new title. In this way, individual volumes can be updated as needed, without having to wait for the completion of all volumes in an edition, and the individual volumes will have a greater identity as independent books.

CPHSL will appear in eight volumes. The editors or authors of each volume are noted below:

Volume 1: Reference and Information Services in Health Sciences Libraries, *M. Sandra Wood, editor*

Volume 2: Educational Services in Health Sciences Libraries, *Francesca Allegri, editor*

Volume 3: Information Access and Delivery in Health Sciences Libraries, *Carolyn E. Lipscomb, editor*

Volume 4: Collection Development and Assessment in Health Sciences Libraries, *by Daniel T. Richards and Dottie Eakin*

Volume 5: Acquisitions in Health Sciences Libraries, *David Morse, editor*

Volume 6: Organization and Management of Information Resources in Health Sciences Libraries, *Laurie L. Thompson, editor*

Volume 7: Health Sciences Environment and Librarianship in Health Sciences Libraries, *Lucretia W. McClure, editor*

Volume 8: Administration and Management in Health Sciences Libraries, *Rick B. Forsman, editor*

The editor-in-chief is extremely fortunate in being able to tap the expertise of a group of very talented and dedicated MLA members as advisors, editors, and chapter authors. The *CPHSL* Advisory Committee provided valuable advice on the organization and content of *CPHSL*, recommended a publication plan and timetable, and assisted in the identification of editors and chapter authors.

The editors have total responsibility for the preparation for publication of their volume, including selection of authors, review of content and adherence to established style and format guidelines, and maintenance of the publication schedule. Authors were asked to include in their chapters, as applicable, the following considerations: ethics, standards, legal aspects, staffing issues and implications, differing practices as they apply to different types of libraries, research, evaluation, technology/automation, and budgeting and financing.

An extensive expert review process involves both academic and hospital librarians. Each volume includes a listing of the expert reviewers in grateful acknowledgement of their efforts. The editor-in-chief and the editors are indebted to MLA's Managing Editor of Books, J. Michael Homan, for selecting reviewers and coordinating their work, and for his personal suggestions on organization, content, and format.

CPHSL is co-published by the Medical Library Association and Scarecrow Press, Inc. Special thanks are due to David B. Biesel, Director of Scarecrow's Association Publishing Program, Raymond S. Naegele, MLA's Director of Financial and Administrative Services, Kimberly S. Pierceall, MLA's Director of Communications, for their advice and assistance. The indexing expertise of Beryl Glitz provides consistent and accurate access to the content of each volume.

Alison Bunting, Editor-in-Chief
Louise M. Darling Biomedical Library
University of California, Los Angeles

Bibliography

1. Doe J, Ed. Handbook of medical library practice. Chicago: American Library Association, 1942: v.

2. Doe J, Marshall, ML, eds. Handbook of medical library practice. 2nd ed. Chicago: American Library Association, 1956.

3. Annan GL, Felter JW, eds. Handbook of medical library practice. 3rd ed. Chicago: Medical Library Association, 1970: v.

4. Ibid., vii.

5. Darling L, Bishop D, Colaianni LA, eds. Handbook of medical library practice. 4th ed. vol. 1. Chicago: Medical Library Association, 1982: xi.

6. Ibid., xi.

7. Ibid., xii.

8. Darling L, Bishop D, Colaianni LA, eds. Handbook of medical library practice. 4th ed. vol. 3. Chicago: Medical Library Association, 1988: xiv.

9. Ibid., xiv.

10. Ibid., xv.

Expert Reviewers

Ysabel R. Bertolucci, Oakland, CA
Virginia M. Bowden, San Antonio, TX
Suzanne K. Dankert, Kalamazoo, MI
Rosalind F. Dudden, Denver, CO
Lelde B. Gilman, Portland, OR
Linda Hulbert, St. Louis, MO
Brenda Lucas, Boston, MA
Anne M. Pascarelli, Boston, MA
Suzanne Porter, Durham, NC
Arlene McFarlin Weismantel, Rochester, MN

Advisory Committee Members

J. Michael Homan
Director of Libraries
Mayo Foundation
Rochester, MN

Mary Horres
Associate University Librarian for Sciences
Biomedical Library
University of California, San Diego
La Jolla, CA

Kimberly Pierceall
Director of Communications
Medical Library Association
Chicago, IL

M. Sandra Wood
Librarian, Reference and Database Services
George T. Harrell Library
Milton S. Hershey Medical Center
Pennsylvania State University
Hershey, PA

Acknowledgments

Many people have had a hand in the preparation of this book. We extend our gratitude to Alison Bunting, Editor-in-Chief of *Current Practice in Health Sciences Librarianship*, and J. Michael Homan, MLA's Managing Editor of Books, for shepherding us through multiple sets of manuscript pages. Thanks also to the expert reviewers named elsewhere who provided fine and incisive commentary, improving several sections and chapters significantly. Appreciation is extended both to MLA for permission to include policy excerpts from MLA DocKit No. 3 [1] and to the unnamed authors of those policies. Acknowledgment is made to librarians in the following libraries for granting permission to reproduce complete institutional collection development policies or significant sections therefrom.

Long Beach Community Hospital Library, Long Beach, CA
Burlew Medical Library, St. Joseph Hospital, Orange, CA
Medical Library, Southern Illinois University, Springfield, IL
Babson Medical Library, Newton-Wellesley Hospital, Newton Lower
    Falls, MA
William H. Welch Medical Library, Johns Hopkins University,
    Baltimore, MD
Maine Medical Center Library, Portland, ME
Biomedical Libraries, Dartmouth College, Hanover, NH
Augustus C. Long Health Sciences Library, Columbia University, New
    York, NY
College of Physicians of Philadelphia Library, Philadelphia, PA
Scott Memorial Library, Thomas Jefferson University, Philadelphia, PA
Houston Academy of Medicine - Texas Medical Center Library,
    Houston, TX
Columbia Hospital Medical Library, Milwaukee, WI

A special note of gratitude goes to Lucretia McClure for permission to use a paper on selection for preservation which she co-authored and which formed the basis for Chapter 11, Preservation [2], and to Terry Ryan for many of the ideas in the budget preparation section of Chapter 8, Budgeting for Collection Development.

Finally, we express our appreciation to Richard A. Tucker, Dana Biomedical Library, Dartmouth College, and to Stacie Husak, Medical Sciences Library, Texas A&M University, who provided invaluable support in the preparation of the manuscript.

Daniel T. Richards
Dottie Eakin

References

1. Morse DH, Richards DT. Collection development policies for health sciences libraries. Chicago: Medical Library Association, 1992. (MLA DocKit No. 3).

2. Richards DT, McClure LW. Selection for preservation: considerations for the health sciences. Bull Med Libr Assoc 1989 Jul; 77(3):284-92.

Introduction

Collection development as a discrete specialized function in health sciences libraries is a relatively recent phenomenon, the term having come into common usage only in the late 1970s. In academic libraries the term has been in use at least since the 1950s and in public libraries a few years prior to that. Broadus, in what he describes as "a tangled skein of ideas, theories, issues, and practices," traces the history of collection development from the Sumerians to the present, noting that over the ages, it is surprising how "uniform the ideas about collection development have been." He goes on to note that collection development in recent times can be characterized as "the continuing refinement of theory, the more skillful organization of personnel and processes, and....model[ling] library selection decision making along clearly rational lines" [1]. There is much about collection development that is common in all types of libraries, and though his context was collection development generally, Broadus' observations are germane to health sciences libraries.

Library collections in health sciences settings have of course been "developed" since the first medical library was founded, and over time there has been a progressive maturation of the process which has as its end result the library collection. Until the decade of the 1970s, however, selection activities in health sciences libraries were usually subsumed under the title "acquisitions librarian" or were regarded as the exclusive province of the library director. However, collection development became the preferred descriptor for this professional specialization in health sciences libraries when the acquisitions process was refined to distinguish selection from procurement, the attentions of the director were turned to other matters, and finally, other tasks such as resource sharing, library user relations, and other collection-related responsibilities were combined with selection.

As health sciences librarians took a more systematized approach to the development of library collections, they paid greater attention to the assessment and evaluation of those collections. Periodic assessments of collections were conducted in some libraries, but this practice was not commonplace. Collection assessment examines through careful planning and analysis the results of collection development activity.

This volume introduces and defines the documentation and decision making processes in collection development, explores organizational models for collection development in health sciences libraries, and describes the rationales and methodologies for assessing health sciences library collections. It also explores the relationship of collection development and assessment to other library functions and services, and addresses the budgeting process. The volume does not cover the technical and business aspects of acquisition and control of library materials. (For information on acquisitions, refer to Volume 5 in this series, *Acquisitions in Health Sciences Libraries.*)

This work is intended for librarians in all types of health sciences libraries, but the principles and topics covered will have application in science libraries as well. The volume may be useful in courses in medical librarianship or in collection development.

Health sciences librarians in all types of settings are charged with the development of a library collection. To be effective in performing this activity, many rely on experience, colleagues, and continuing education (CE) courses to acquire and maintain their skills. There are few who leave their graduate education with more than a basic understanding of the principles of collection development. Several recent books [2-5] cover the principles of collection development generally or in academic and research libraries, and the American Library Association (ALA) has introduced a useful series of pamphlets, *Collection Management and Development Guides* [6], which provide concise coverage of the fundamentals of specific collection development routines such as drafting a policy statement. There is no comparable work on collection development for health sciences librarians, though there are related chapters in earlier editions of the *Handbook of Medical Library Practice* [7], in *Hospital Library Management* [8], and in other books on health sciences librarianship. There are also important articles on collection development topics in the *Bulletin of the Medical Library Association* and other library science periodicals.

Our aim has not been to prepare a comprehensive work on collection development itself, but rather to provide a text that describes the application of collection development principles in health sciences libraries. In one sense this volume is a compilation of relevant material from the vast literature related to collection development, compiled so that the reader can find in a single source some appropriate guidance for collection development in medical settings. In another sense, it is our attempt to relay to others, in a systematic fashion, our experience in collection development in a range of libraries over the past twenty-five years. For that reason, the text may reflect an academic library perspective more often than a hospital or special library view. The principles of collection development apply equally as well in all types of health sciences libraries and we feel that librarians in settings other than academic health sciences libraries can find value in this book.

The collection development process is taking place more and more in a rapidly changing environment, and the material presented here will change to reflect that environment. The very character of collections in health sciences libraries is being altered as we attempt to accommodate access and ownership, to incorporate with print materials information in a bewildering array of electronic formats, and to educate library users about the fundamental importance of information in the health care enterprise. The reader is advised to maintain an awareness of changes in collection development and to apply those changes as appropriate.

Errors, however unintentional, will be found in this text; we assume full responsibility for them, and expect readers to point them out to us. Readers too will take issue with some of our interpretations, recommendations, and guidance; that is the nature of things. Ultimately, it is the reader who will determine how well we have achieved our goal of closing a gap in the literature of collection development and health sciences librarianship.

Daniel T. Richards
Dottie Eakin

References

1. Broadus RN. The history of collection development. In: Osburn CB, Atkinson R, eds. Collection management: a new treatise. Greenwich, CT: JAI Press, 1991:22. (Foundations in library and information science, v. 26A).

2. Magrill RM, Hickey DJ. Acquisitions management and collection development in libraries. 2d ed. Chicago: American Library Association, 1989.

3. Osburn CB, Atkinson R, eds. Collection management: a new treatise. Greenwich, CT: JAI Press, 1991. (Foundations in library and information science, v. 26A-B).

4. Sellen BC, Curley A. The collection building reader. New York: Neal-Schuman, 1992.

5. Wortman WA. Collection management: background and principles. Chicago: American Library Association, 1989.

6. American Library Association. Association for Library Collections and Technical Services. Collection management and development guides, no. 1- . Chicago: American Library Association, 1989- .

7. Eakin D. Health science library materials: collection development. In: Darling L, Bishop D, Colaianni LA, eds. Handbook of medical library practice. 4th ed. v.2. Chicago: Medical Library Association, 1989:27-91.

8. Hardy MC. Selection of library materials. In: Bradley J, Holst R, Messerle J, eds. Hospital library management. Chicago: Medical Library Association, 1983:29-44.

The Context for Collection Development in Health Sciences Libraries

"As a rule, disease can scarcely keep pace with the itch to scribble about it."
John Mayow,
Tractatus duo, 1668

"The proportion of what is both new and true is not much greater in medicine than it is in theology."
John Shaw Billings,
Transactions of the American Association of Physicians, 1891

The library's collection is its heart because it is the collection that is the central information resource upon which most library activities rely. The traditional concept of a library is one of a collection of books, periodicals, newspapers, pamphlets and other materials kept for reading, reference, or circulation. Today's vision of the collection must incorporate both a broader range of materials, especially to include those in electronic and other nonbook forms, and a greater sense of connectivity, to include access to resources external to the physical place. A library is also a physical place in which the business of information occurs, whether through the intermediary of the library staff or by direct action of a library user.

It is the development of a health sciences library's collection that is the focus of this volume—how materials for it are identified, selected, organized, preserved; who the principal players are; how the collection reflects the institution of which it is a part; how the effectiveness of the collection is assessed; and related topics. The library's collection in the aggregate is ultimately a selection from a vast universe of information on medical and related subjects.

It is beyond the scope of this volume to provide an in-depth analysis of the biomedical literature or to describe in detail the variations among and between the literatures of individual biomedical subjects and disciplines. There is a very large bibliography of readily available books and periodical articles which address these topics. This chapter provides a short introduction to the biomedical literature through a discussion of publication patterns, literature types, growth rates, and the scholarly record of biomedicine. Information is also included concerning the collection of the National Library of Medicine (NLM), the largest of its kind and one which defines the universe of biomedical literature insofar as a library collection can do so. The chapter concludes with a brief essay on the evolution of collection development in health sciences libraries. Together, these two parts form a context for the remainder of the volume.

The Role of the Biomedical Literature

The primary role of the literature of a scientific discipline is to record and transmit discoveries and ideas which advance the state of knowledge within that discipline. At its most basic, this role can be defined as communication and is made manifest through publication of information. Publishing and scientific communication have been intertwined virtually since the issuance of the first scientific periodical in the seventeenth century.

Another function of scientific literature is to help solve problems in research or practice; the ability to do so is directly affected by the amount and quality of relevant information available to support those activities. Still other functions are to assign primacy of discovery, to support promotion and tenure, to maintain a permanent record of scientific accomplishment, and to provide justification for the grant seeking process.

As communication patterns among scientists change, traditional publication patterns also change. The principal change in communication now is engendered by the ubiquitous personal workstation and its networking capabilities. Additional influences include ready access to telecommunication networks and the transfer of information in unreviewed form. Ironically, the computer coupled with word processing technology has resulted in a greater ability to produce manuscripts, adding in large measure to the flood of material.

There are differences between the publication patterns of scientists and of humanists. Humanists and scientists are divided not only by their lingua franca but also by the form their work takes; humanists primarily write books but scientists primarily write articles, largely because of the rapid pace of scientific discovery and the requirement that results be published and communicated quickly. There is also some feeling that the level of specialization in the sciences minimizes the potential number of readers and thus, book buyers, which makes scientific book publishing a more risky economic enterprise. The obsolescence of information by the time it is published contributes to the publishing risk factor in rapidly moving fields of medicine.

The biomedical literature contains vast amounts of information, some of which is important and original, more that is mundane and repetitive. "Value resides not in the literature but in the consensus of ideas that experienced scientists create out of it" [1]. Scientific literature can also be regarded metaphorically as a form of external memory from which we can extract and add at will. One may also view it as a structure made up of additions of small segments until a larger picture emerges. Ortega y Gasset postulates that "science advances by many small discoveries" [2].

The biomedical literature then can be viewed structurally in many different ways: by format, by subject, by date, by country of origin, by publisher, by language, or other perspective. One or more of these structural views can have utility in collection development generally and is frequently a prominent feature in policy statements. The rising availability of information in electronic formats, such as preprints, current awareness resources, structural data and graphics, presents new challenges to librarians in collection development. The definition of "literature" must incorporate these new formats as well.

The principal challenge of collection development is to explore the biomedical literature in its broadest interpretation and to determine which segments or pieces of that literature are most appropriate to support the information needs of the group of users associated with the library. A comprehensive knowledge of the way literature is structured and how it changes is not necessary for success in collection development, but there are several aspects of it that can inform the decision making processes of collection development.

Types of Literature and Their Importance

As noted, the structure of the literature is important to consider. Importance indicators may be assigned to major portions of the literature and librarians use these distinctions as guides in collection development. There are, for example, three principal levels of materials, each by its name reflecting in a real sense the relative importance of that level to biomedical literature as a whole. These three levels are

> **PRIMARY** level material, which includes source documents, such as journals, monographs, treatises, manuscripts, patient records, prints and portraits, and collateral reference items that contain original observations, annotated bibliographies, dictionaries;
> **SECONDARY** level material, which includes reviews, state-of-the-art summaries, textbooks, interpretations of primary sources, conclusions derived from primary sources;
> **TERTIARY** level material, which includes the remainder of the synthetic literature, or repackaging of the primary literature for a purpose other than that intended by the author, such as popular treatments, annuals, handbooks, and encyclopedias.

Among the considerations that are evident from the descriptions of the levels for collection development decision making are the degree of importance of each level to the range of clinical, research, or educational activity supported by the library collection. In general, the greater the research effort the more the library should collect primary level materials. Similarly, the collection that primarily supports an education program will have a higher need for secondary and tertiary level material.

Another way to analyze the literature is to divide it by format, such as serials and books. Under each of these a determination of primary, secondary, tertiary can be made, as follows:

> **PRIMARY** serial sources include journals containing original peer-reviewed articles and aimed at a general or specialist audience;
> **SECONDARY** serial sources include those which publish review articles, summaries of current opinion, news items;
> **TERTIARY** serial sources include indexes and abstracts and other similar guides to other serial literature [3].

It is generally acknowledged that the journal literature represents the most important format of the published literature of biomedicine, with books assuming a subordinate place in the literature. Periodicals and journals are resources published at regular intervals which contain original articles reporting general or specialized research information, review articles, current opinion, and the like. This type of publication is most useful for state-of-the-art research data and specialized clinical case information. The periodical review literature, which synthesizes and typically evaluates in a single location information from a wide range of sources, was once regarded as redundant but was collected for its convenience. This type of literature is assuming greater importance in library collections as it takes on an increased role as a current awareness and quality filtering tool.

Specific book formats play different roles in conveying information as well. Textbooks, monographs, and other definitive publications present an array of information about a topic or a field, in a convenient single volume format. These works typically synthesize material from other sources, particularly periodicals. Books are most useful for factual data, descriptive summaries and overviews, historical information, and in-depth information.

Libraries frequently make collecting distinctions between types of books, especially between textbooks and monographs. Textbook editions are generally published in larger press runs that are intended to be superseded by later editions. They most often are general treatments of a discipline and lack the depth and detail of a monograph. Most textbooks are based on the premise that education is a continuous process and are written with that in mind. For example, textbooks are frequently prepared to be definitive for teaching purposes, but not for the discipline. Consequently, textbooks have a shorter life, affected by trends in education, by the popularity of teaching methods, and by the changing importance of disciplines.

Monographs, by contrast, may be described as "ageless" [4] and they most frequently contain a thorough presentation on a narrow subject. They generally have a permanent usefulness in a library, especially because subsequent authors may not undertake the same type of intensive review. An attempt to be comprehensive within a restricted area underlies the preparation of a monograph. One might observe that, in general, the more specific and more specialized the topic, the longer the book is likely to be valuable in a library collection. Books in specialties are generally felt to have a longer life than general titles, though those not regarded as classics may quickly become obsolete, especially in highly technical and rapidly advancing fields such as radiology. As more and more library collections become client-oriented, or as the focus in selection is on expressed need, the place of the monograph in the collection will diminish.

The visual record too is of great importance in the biomedical literature and it is present in both journals and monographs in the form of plates, portraits, photomicrographs, and radiographs. Visual representations constitute an integral part of the literature of medicine and may indeed be each worth a thousand words, because they alone, or in sequence, may form the very essence of an article. The visual record assumes a greater importance in digital form as librarians witness the rise of structural biochemistry, visual comparisons in which scientists search for homologies, and structural cell biology. Only in art is the visual as important to the scholarly record.

Aural or visual presentations also appear in a wide variety of formats, such as audiotapes, videotapes, and slides, or in formats that combine media. These may be produced in series or as stand-alone publications and are most useful for explanations of complex procedures, hard-to-describe sounds, or situations such as role playing and patient education, in which multiple factors are important and not evident in written formats.

Distribution and Size of the Scholarly Record

The scholarly record of biomedicine is immense. The collection of the NLM holds more than 2 million book items, and another 3 million nonbook items. These figures include more than 675,000 monographs, approximately 1,000,000 periodical volumes, 300,000 historical theses, 172,000 pamphlets, and approximately 55,000 audiovisual items. NLM maintains approximately 23,000 subscriptions and more than 185,000 pieces arrive annually.

The Library of Congress (LC) and the National Agricultural Library (NAL) each have collections in the health sciences, significant portions of which duplicate those at NLM. Unique collections in the health sciences include LC's coverage of the popular medical literature and its comprehensive collections of related subjects such as anthropology and biology. The vast LC collections in psychology and sociology are becoming more important to the health sciences as health care practice changes to a more comprehensive view of the patient. NAL collects some areas of veterinary medicine more comprehensively than NLM, and houses large collections of relevant government publications, legislation, and foreign government reports that are complementary to those held at NLM.

Beyond NLM and the other national libraries, there is a large network of medical libraries, both in the United States and abroad, which hold varying percentages of unique materials. Mammoth collections of records exist outside libraries in museums and archives, in patient-file rooms in medical centers, and in the files of practicing physicians and other health care providers. Actual numbers of items in each category are impossible to estimate as national inventories have not been done. Despite the imprecision in the last category, however, the numbers are significant, and all of these collections combined result in a scholarly record for biomedicine which comprises many millions of items. NLM itself recognizes that the scholarly record of biomedicine is distributed as the following illustrates.

The centrality of the NLM collection to the concept of a national collection in biomedicine and the complementary nature of other library collections is well recognized. NLM, in its 1986 Long Range

Plan describes a distributed library of record for the biomedical sciences and acknowledges that "even within any narrowly identified scope of biomedical materials, there is more than any single library can acquire." Indeed, among the Nation's biomedical libraries are many collections of unique materials.

The national collection in any discipline, therefore, is not limited to the holdings of a single national library, nor is it simply the sum of all titles within a given subject. It is a composite of individual titles and important special collections located in many different institutions. NLM seeks to identify existing strengths in other collections and to encourage other libraries to collect unique materials, particularly state and local biomedical literature, manuscripts, and items of strong local interest [5].

Growth Rates

De Solla Price plotted growth rates of scientific literature over time and concluded that the literature of most scientific disciplines doubles every fifteen years [6]. This growth rate has been relatively constant across scientific disciplines, including the health sciences. Lock challenged de Solla Price's theory by stating that the so-called "explosion" of literature is an illusion. He suggested that in fact the rate of expansion of the literature has been relatively constant at 5-7% per year [7]. There is truth in each theory because each author justifies his view by examining the growth process from different perspectives. De Solla Price examines all literature while Lock examines what he regards as the core periodical literature of various disciplines.

A more recent study of the periodicals collection of the National Library of Medicine shows that since the 1850s, there has been a slow but steady increase in the number of new publications over the last 135 years; this rise reached a peak in the 1950s, declined through the 1960s and 1970s, and rose slowly through the 1980s [8]. Whichever measuring stick one uses, the growth rate for the literature of biomedicine is significant and is something of particular importance to collection development because it is from this universe that library collections are selected. Fortunately, there is also a significantly high death rate for the health sciences literature. Periodicals cease to be published and books become obsolete.

Factors affecting growth rates of the scientific literature include the increasing cost of science, especially for instrumentation, the degree of specialization leading to fragmentation of disciplines, and the converse, an increase in interdisciplinary approaches to scientific disciplines. The changing standards for publication coupled with an increased number of writers generating documents for publishing will affect the number of items being published, as do technological changes that have made document generation so easy, such as word processing software and desk-top publishing. The continued growth in the number of publishable articles and the increased size of journal issues are frequently cited by journal publishers as justification for constantly rising prices.

Growth of the Periodical Literature

In 1800, there were approximately ninety scientific journals being published. By 1900, that figure had risen to more than 10,000. In 1994, there were more than 35,000 active periodical publications in the health sciences. As noted, the growth rate for health sciences titles peaked in the 1950s and declined through the next two decades. In the 1980s the downward trend reversed and is slowly rising once again [9].

The principal reasons for starting new health sciences journals include both the splintering of disciplines and the opposite phenomenon—the interdisciplinary approach to a subject. Other reasons are to enhance communication or stimulate research within a discipline, to educate health professionals, or to provide a common forum to consolidate material of interest that is scattered in a variety of publications. Still other journals are brought into existence in connection with an organization or an association of individuals with common interests. Additional reasons include the need to stimulate research in the discipline, to synthesize or review the recent literature; to educate professionals, to improve patient care, to publish abstracts or proceedings, to meet the need for an "international," "American," or "European" journal in the discipline, and, of course, the profit motive.

SERHOLD contains nearly 40,000 records, reflecting principally active titles, but also including some titles in disciplines outside the health sciences. CATLINE contains some 70,000 serial records of all types, demonstrating that there are approximately as many dead titles as live ones. King, McDonald, and Roderer [10] demonstrated that the number of articles grows at a rate relatively parallel to journal title growth. The proliferation of journals led to the development of abstracting and indexing services, which have grown at a rate of about one for each 300 new journals. The growth rate for journals in the United States has been very rapid but slightly slower than the worldwide rate.

Growth rates for periodicals at the discipline level are difficult to determine because no comprehensive study has been undertaken. Subject lists of journals prepared by periodical vendors are common, as are subject studies at the specialty or discipline level and of periodicals indexed in

Index Medicus. Among the best of the *Index Medicus* subject-based studies is the one prepared by EBSCO [11]. *Current Contents,* published by the Institute for Scientific Information, has carried for many years the occasional insightful analysis of the periodicals in individual specialties.

Growth of the Book Literature

The expansion in publication rates for monographs, textbooks, treatises, and book literature in the health sciences also is significant. Many of the reasons for publication of books parallel those for periodicals. Books are published in response to subdivision of specialties and to provide an interdisciplinary approach to a topic. Books provide a convenient mechanism for consolidation of discipline-based information that appears in many publications. There is a steady flow of monographs on more and more specialized topics and of textbooks to meet the needs of classroom and continuing education for the health professional. Organizations and associations often have aggressive publishing programs to respond to their membership, and numerous new publications are issued by federal, state, and local governments.

Figures for the monograph literature are less precise than figures for the periodical literature, but NLM's collection contains at least 675,000 books. Though the collection is comprehensive, there are, in several other libraries, substantial collections that do not duplicate those at NLM. If one estimates that figure to be in the neighborhood of 25%, the health sciences monograph literature may well reach 850,000. Other types of book literature including theses, reports, pamphlets, documents, and other nonserial publications, taken together would suggest a number nearly equal that.

Annually, the U.S. book trade produces approximately 3,500 new medical books, including some English language imports [12]. Worldwide, there are many more books published, however, as demonstrated by NLM's acquisitions figures for books, which show that about 15,000 books are added annually [13].

Analyzed at the discipline level, however, these gross figures show that the book literature of some fields is much larger than others and that subfields of medicine have widely varying growth rates. Table 1-1 presents data about the relative sizes of the subject universes for books based on a review of CATLINE records. It also shows for the period 1985-1994 the publication rates for those same groupings, as represented by book trade statistics provided by Ballen Booksellers International [14]. These figures are not absolutes because they do not take into account all of the world's book production. Because they are based on reliable sources, however, they provide a picture of the way in which the monograph literature of medicine

Table 1-1: Health Sciences Books

(NLM Collection Figures by Subject from CATLINE, March, 1995;
Book Publishing 1985-94 from Ballen Booksellers International)

NLM Class	Subject	NLM Holdings 1995	Books Published 1985-94	Annual Growth Rate Bks/Yr
	Preclinical Sciences			
QS	Anatomy	6,295	356	36
QT	Physiology	10,289	751	75
QU	Biochemistry	10,855	1,311	131
QV	Pharmacology	23,508	1,284	128
QW	Microbiology/Immunology	8,710	1,189	119
QX	Parasitology	1,983	74	7
QY	Clinical Pathology	4,962	251	25
QZ	Pathology	11,142	1,098	110
	SUBTOTALS	77,744	6,314	
	Medicine			
W	Medical Profession	27,062	2,353	235
WA	Public Health	26,498	1,305	130
WB	Practice of Medicine	25,901	996	100
WC	Communicable Diseases	11,133	388	39
WD	Nutrition, Metabolic & Immunologic Diseases	6,020	583	58
WE	Musculoskeletal System	13,680	1,318	132
WF	Respiratory System	8,627	515	52
WG	Cardiovascular System	12,976	1,270	127
WH	Hemic/Lymphatic System	4,866	337	34
WI	Gastrointestinal System	10,298	712	71
WJ	Urogenital System	6,412	547	55
WK	Endocrine System	5,913	484	48
WL	Nervous System	17,079	2,115	212
WM	Psychiatry	32,554	3,083	308
WN	Radiology	6,983	453	45
WO	Surgery	11,602	1,088	109
WP	Gynecology	8,299	611	61
WQ	Obstetrics	7,899	566	57
WR	Dermatology	4,400	301	30
WS	Pediatrics	16,212	1,398	140
WT	Geriatrics	4,498	316	32
WU	Dentistry	9,597	594	59
WV	Otorhinolaryngology	5,239	378	38
WW	Ophthalmology	8,574	638	64
WX	Hospitals	11,612	334	33
WY	Nursing	13,395	1,367	137
WZ	History of Medicine	46,981	263	26
	SUBTOTALS	364,310	24,313	
	TOTALS	442,054	30,627	

is divided in the largest medical library in the world and how those divisions have grown during the past decade.

In the preclinical sciences the annual growth rate ranges from seven new titles per year in parasitology to 131 for the faster growing and larger field of biochemistry. By contrast, many clinical fields grow at much higher rates; the field of psychiatry, for example, has grown at a rate of approximately 300 titles per year since 1985. Human anatomy by contrast grows at an even slower rate of fewer than forty titles per year, not too surprising since the subject matter is relatively constant. These variations reflect the proportionate differences between the basic sciences and clinical disciplines, the different levels of research activity among medical specialties, and other factors such as the age of the discipline and the number of practitioners and researchers it claims. These figures can be useful in budget planning, collection assessment, and preservation.

Guides to the Literature

In addition to the general publishing and book trade publications such as *Ulrich's International Periodicals Directory, The Serials Directory, Books in Print*, and other Bowker products such as *Medical Books and Periodicals in Print*, there are many useful guides to the biomedical literature. These guides provide information on publishing trends and recommendations for specific titles, as well as fundamental information about biomedical specialties. This type of publication can play a key role in collection development and assessment in any type of health sciences library. It is good practice for those carrying out the functions of collection development to become familiar with bibliographies, subject guides, lists of periodicals, and other publications of this type. The knowledge will be important in virtually any collection development activity.

A very useful resource is Morton and Godbolt's *Information Sources in the Medical Sciences*, presently in its fourth edition [15]. Though many of its references are to British publications, this guide contains informative chapters on the different types of biomedical literature and their place in library collections, followed by a series of chapters on the literatures of medical disciplines and specialties. Each chapter is written by a subject expert who discusses and recommends textbooks, periodicals, reference works, historical resources, and works at the subspecialty level. It also includes a good introduction to historical, biographical, and bibliographical sources in biomedicine.

Haselbauer's *A Research Guide to the Health Sciences: Medical, Nutritional and Environmental* [16], is a well-organized evaluative guide to information sources in biomedicine. Despite its inclusion in a series called "Reference

Sources for the Social Sciences and Humanities," it provides, in bibliographic essay form, sections on general works arranged by type, the basic sciences, and the social aspects of the health sciences, with the bulk of the book devoted to chapters on medical specialties.

"Core" lists, or highly selective guides to the literature, can be very helpful tools to the librarian selecting items for a library collection. Those developed by Brandon and Hill [17-19] are especially well known and regarded as primary selection tools in most health sciences libraries. The most popular is the "Selected List of Books and Journals for the Small Medical Library" which began in 1965 and has been updated approximately every two years since. It offers a recommended list of books and periodicals, organized primarily by subject, and is designed as a selection guide for small and medium-size health sciences libraries. A new feature since the fifteenth edition in 1993 is the inclusion of a "minimal core list" chosen from the overall list. Another well-received list is the "Library for Internists" [20] which appears in *Annals of Internal Medicine* approximately every three years. There are lists prepared for many disciplines that can be useful as checklists for collection development and assessment in those fields.

Collection Development in Health Sciences Libraries

As the introduction to this volume states, collection development as a discrete specialized function in health sciences libraries is a relatively recent phenomenon, though the concept and the rubric have been generally employed in academic libraries for some time. The terms "collection development" and "collection development officer" had their origins in academe and were first used in health sciences libraries in the late 1970s. Prior to that time, selection activities in medical libraries were typically carried out by an "acquisitions librarian" or the library director.

Health sciences librarians have, of course, been developing collections since the establishment of the first medical library; but in the last fifteen years or so, the processes, policies, and philosophies surrounding that activity have been scrutinized and articulated in such a way that a new specialty has arisen. Hill traced the development of health sciences librarianship's newest specialty at the inaugural lecture of MLA's Collection Development Round Table in 1983 and observed that "the library collection is the foundation upon which all other library services are dependent." She extended that reasoning to conclude that "developing the collection is one of the most important—if not *the* most important—of pursuits in librarianship" [21].

Several factors contributed to the evolution of collection development as it is known today. The distinction between the two principal aspects of "acquisitions"—selection and procurement—was reinforced by the usual assignment of responsibility for the former to the library director or a portion of the user group, especially the faculty in academic settings. The acquisitions librarian was more of an order librarian and the professional literature of acquisitions in large measure focused on procedures and detail. As institutions became more complex and the attention of the administrator and faculty was taken by other tasks, responsibility for selection ultimately was vested in the acquisitions librarian. Budgets began to tighten as the output from the publishing industry began to escalate exponentially, making selection a more complex task. Documentation of selection principles led to the more systematic codification of overall policies and procedures, as well as the expansion of responsibilities regarded as selection related. The broadening of responsibilities led to the use of the term "collection development." Today, collection development in many libraries embraces a wide variety of functions.

Collection development librarians in health sciences institutions frequently assume responsibility for selection as well as other functions such as budget planning, resource sharing, and collection management. These activities, which are not necessarily new but may be newly emphasized, span the traditional technical services and public services division within most libraries. Success in collection development requires a sophisticated understanding of the health care professions, as well as a solid knowledge of the creation and use of health sciences literature and information. This knowledge has, in most instances, been acquired through experience rather than through formal library school or continuing education activities.

Eakin demonstrates that expenditures for the acquisition of books, journals, and audiovisual materials are exceeded in most library budgets only by those for personnel, and shows that just as a substantial reference staff does not assure good service, neither does generous funding for materials guarantee a good quality collection [22]. Minimal support for a collection more frequently results in a poor quality collection. A library's collections should be developed in a manner consistent with its overall goals, and collection development implies not only the selection of specific materials but also a master plan—a vision of how the library, responding to its unique set of circumstances and responsibilities, will build its collections and make the wisest use of its resources.

Hospital Libraries

Collection development in hospital libraries is not dramatically different from collection development in academic or other types of medical libraries, though some important distinctions can be drawn. The hospital librarian generally has a keener knowledge of the library's collection as well as a more detailed knowledge of the user group. There is a substantial difference usually in the level of financial resources available for collection development and there is a greater reliance on resource sharing in responding to information needs of the user group. Brandon and Hill [23] have observed that collection development in hospital settings is different because errors in selection are relatively more costly and certainly more obvious than in a large medical center library. Hospital libraries tend also to have a greater involvement of library users in the selection process, frequently in the form of a library committee that provides input to a process coordinated by the librarian. An intimate knowledge of the clinical and research programs of the hospital is critical to the process.

Basic Functions of Collection Development

The five basic functions of collection development include the identification of literature, the selection of literature, deselection or withdrawal of literature, preservation of the literature, and evaluation or collection assessment. Other functions include budgeting and budget projection, policy writing and documentation, report generation, and analysis of the literature.

Libraries exist within an institutional context and the purposes of the institution and the library's user groups need to be identified and kept at the forefront of the collection development process. The goals of the library must be connected to the goals of the institution. Health sciences library collections, in general, are developed to support one or more of five basic activities within that institution. These include clinical practice and health care services; research by faculty, staff, and students; education and training of health care professionals; administration of health care services and educational programs; and, to a lesser degree than the others, the preservation of institutional publications or related materials. This chapter has introduced the broad spectrum of collection development principles in health sciences libraries. Subsequent chapters will expand on the application of these principles.

References

1. Dannatt RJ. Primary sources of information. In: Morton LT, Godbolt S, eds. Information sources in the medical sciences. 4th ed. London: Bowker-Saur, 1992:25.

2. Ortega y Gasset J. Revolt of the masses. New York: Norton, 1932:34.

3. Mathews DA, Picken F. Medical librarianship. London: Bingley, 1979.

4. Crawford H. Treasure or white elephant? Bull Med Libr Assoc 1970 Jul;58(3):336-40.

5. Collection development manual of the National Library of Medicine. 3rd ed. Bethesda, MD: National Library of Medicine, 1993:5-6.

6. De Solla Price D. Little science, big science. New York: Columbia University Press, 1963:39.

7. Lock S. "Journalology"—are the quotes needed? CBE Views 1989 Aug;12(2):57.

8. Humphreys BL, McCutcheon DE. Growth patterns in the National Library of Medicine's serials collection and in Index Medicus journals, 1966-1985. Bull Med Libr Assoc 1994 Jan;82(1):18-24.

9. Ibid., 21.

10. King DW, McDonald DD, Roderer NK. Scientific journals in the United States: their production, use and economics. Stroudsburg, PA: Hutchinson Ross, 1981.

11. Fortney LM, Basile VA. Index Medicus price study. Birmingham, AL: EBSCO, 1996.

12. Bowker Annual of Library and Book Trade Information. New York: Bowker, 1979- .

13. National Library of Medicine. Programs & services. Fiscal year. Bethesda, MD: National Library of Medicine, 1977- .

14. Schrift L, Moran L. Ten-year NLM cumulative title-price analysis. Hauppauge, NY: Ballen Booksellers International, 1995.

15. Morton LT, Godbolt S, eds. Information sources in the medical sciences. 4th ed. London: Bowker-Saur, 1992.

16. Haselbauer KJ. A research guide to the health sciences: medical, nutritional and environmental. New York: Greenwood Press, 1987. (Reference sources for the social sciences and humanities, no. 4).

17. Brandon AN, Hill DR. Selected list of books and journals for the small medical library. Bull Med Libr Assoc 1995 Apr;83(2):151-75.

18. Brandon AN, Hill DR. Selected list of nursing books and journals. Nurs Outlook 1994 Mar/Apr;42(2):71-82.

19. Brandon AN, Hill DR. Selected list of books and journals in allied health. Bull Med Libr Assoc 1994 Jul;82(3):247-64.

20. Mazza JJ. A library for internists VIII. Recommendations from the American College of Physicians. Ann Intern Med 1994 Apr 15;120(8):699-720.

21. Hill D. The development of collection development in medical libraries. Unpublished paper presented at the Annual Meeting of the Medical Library Association, Houston, TX, May 1983.

22. Eakin D. Health science library materials: collection development. In Darling L, Bishop D, Colaianni LA, eds. Handbook of medical library practice. 4th ed. v.2. Chicago: Medical Library Association, 1989:27.

23. Brandon AN, Hill DR. Selected list of books and journals for the small medical library. Bull Med Libr Assoc 1993 Apr;81(2):141-68.

2

Roles and Relationships in Collection Development

"The drive toward organization is the drive to change everything into means and tools."

Novalis

After setting the context for collection development, the next step is to look at the various functions within the broad set of responsibilities. Who oversees which functions will differ from library to library, but within any one library there must be a clear understanding of where the responsibilities lie. The need to define functions is important even in a small library with one librarian, because that librarian will have a relationship to a committee or administrator and must balance this activity with others.

Some functions encompassed by collection development and management include

- Assessing user needs.
- Coordinating selection activities.
- Developing resource sharing plans.
- Evaluating collections.
- Formulating policies.
- Monitoring and managing expenditures.
- Planning budgets.
- Preserving collections.

- Promoting collection use.
- Selecting books, journals, nonprint resources.
- Training and evaluating selectors.

Organization for Collection Development

Collection development functions have been increasingly formalized in academic libraries since the 1970s [1-4]. The larger the library, the more options one has for organizing collection development functions. Most of the literature related to organizational structure comes out of academic libraries [5-7]. Models may be grouped into two basic types: centralized and decentralized. Each approach has advantages and disadvantages.

Centralized Model

In the centralized model, one person has responsibility for collection development. This person does all the book selection, but may work with a committee or group to select journals and nonprint resources. Budget development, analysis, and monitoring fall within this person's responsibilities, as does collection policy development and any assessment activities.

In a one-librarian library, collection development functions will necessarily fall to that person although an advisory committee is often involved in decision making or approval. Larger libraries have a greater range of choices. Centralizing selection and collection management activities economizes staff time and concentrates knowledge of the collection and control over its growth. The collection development librarian becomes the expert, the one who knows the strengths and weaknesses of the collection in detail, as well as in general—sees both the trees and the forest. Over time, a collection development librarian commands a wealth of critical knowledge about biomedical literature and the library's clientele. The same individual establishes (or at least proposes) policies, selects materials to fulfill needs, and evaluates adequacy of collections. Policies are apt to be applied more consistently. Understanding the broad sweep of biomedical disciplines as well as the scope of publications within those disciplines strengthens the ability to balance the collections to meet the greatest needs of all constituent groups. Budgets can be planned and managed with a more thorough mastery of facts.

A librarian who devotes full-time to collection development activities may have fewer opportunities for contacts with library users. Therefore, where collection development functions are centralized, the librarian must develop and use reliable and efficient methods for soliciting and acquiring information from and about the user community.

Decentralized Model

In this model, selection responsibilities are distributed among several librarians who are generally called selectors or bibliographers and who exercise this collection development assignment along with other job responsibilities. The collection budget for books may also be divided and allocated to selectors, who are given responsibility for managing expenditures within their allocation. A collection development librarian often coordinates selectors' work, may provide training, and in some cases is also responsible for performance review.

While it may be less efficient to distribute the responsibilities among several librarians for selection or evaluation of materials for the collection, the library gains in several ways. Librarians involved in making decisions about the collection will have a far greater appreciation of its content and strengths; as a result they will be better interpreters of the collection. The most common form of decentralization is to divide selection responsibilities by subject. Librarians are often assigned responsibilities on the basis of graduate or professional degrees, past experience, or special interest. The nurse-librarian who selects materials in nursing not only brings a first-hand knowledge of the authors and publications in the field and the current issues, but as a peer of the library's nursing clientele, will have a unique ability to assess needs. Librarians with backgrounds in other health fields or academic training in the life sciences or biotechnology are often especially suited to undertake collection responsibilities. They contribute subject expertise that another individual would not have.

When librarians without special subject knowledge take on collection responsibilities in a specific discipline, they may be motivated to learn more about the field by attending classes, seminars, or conferences, or by reading. In this way they also develop contacts with researchers or practitioners, enhancing their ability to interpret information needs in the field. Regardless of their subject expertise, librarians with public service responsibilities—information services, education, consulting, research support, clinical support, outreach, interlibrary loan, or access services—have well-developed working relationships with library users. They know from reference questions, database searches, library instruction programs, attending rounds, and assisting students with assignments what directions current research is taking, what clinical topics are important, and what is being taught to health professional students. They will become familiar with the important issues in biomedical sciences and health care.

Collection activities may enrich jobs of both public services and technical services librarians, where these traditional divisions remain intact, and contribute to job satisfaction. When both are involved, this structure promotes interaction between divisions within the library.

One disadvantage of the distributed model is that it may not fit well within the traditional hierarchical structure of the library. Reporting lines may be unclear and there may be conflict in priorities between different responsibilities. This topic is discussed more fully in Chapter 3, Education and Training for Collection Development. Because they are concentrating on specific subsets of the collection, individual selectors may not have a comprehensive view of the whole and may be less aware of imbalances than an individual who is overseeing the entire collection. An additional hazard of distributed responsibilities is the potential for selectors to become insular and overprotective of their own assigned areas. A warning from academic libraries: "Subject specialists tend to have highly developed territorial instincts expressed as 'my faculty' or 'my subject' and a much less developed view of the library collections as a whole" [8]. Morse has expressed a skeptical view of delegating collection responsibilities to multiple individuals: "The time spent on selection activities reaches the point of diminishing returns very soon, i.e., that conducting an elaborate, participatory collections development effort results in a collection that is only marginally better—if at all—than a single individual carrying out a basically seat-of-the-pants effort" [9].

Actual Practice

The foregoing are pure models. In truth, hybrids of these types are more common. A study of collection development positions advertised in *College and Research Libraries News* found that 58% were combined positions, with 80% of these involving reference functions. Only 42% were full-time collection development positions [10]. Few health science libraries devote an entire position to collection development and many involve multiple staff to varying degrees in collection development or management responsibilities. An informal survey of collection development staffing patterns conducted of subscribers to the *Biomedical Library Acquisitions Bulletin* turned up a similar variety of organizational structures [11]. Many libraries are undergoing considerable organizational change, leaving the traditional hierarchy behind for greater emphasis on management by teams. The team approach is not new to collection development and fits well into such structures. Each library must determine the structure that will work best.

The institutional setting, the range of talent and interest, and the distribution of other responsibilities will all be factors influencing organization for collection development within the library.

As modern collection development activity emphasizes meeting current needs over building collections for potential future use, those responsible for collections must be in close touch with users. Understanding the institutional environment and the information requirements of the library's constituencies is equally important as knowing the literature. Any model that ignores this element will be deficient.

These models also assume that most collection decisions are made within the library, based on information from, or consultation with, user groups. In practice, especially in smaller libraries, representatives of the user community may have a stronger, if not controlling role, and a committee external to the library may be the primary decision-making body.

Responsibilities

Whatever organizational structure is used, assignments must be clearly defined. Job descriptions should reflect the relative importance of, and anticipated percentage of, time devoted to collection activities. Responsibilities fall into two broad categories: collection development and administration.

Collection Development

The scope of the selector's job should be outlined, including any responsibilities for weeding, collection evaluation, preservation, policy formulation, fund management, and coordination with other libraries. The degree of responsibility and authority to make decisions should also be clearly stated. Expectations of and relationships to other individuals or units should be made clear. Even if collection-related responsibilities are a small proportion of an individual's job, they should be addressed in periodic goal setting and performance evaluation.

Administration

Both the library director and the collection development administrator (if the library has one) have responsibilities for budget management and professional development. The director has ultimate fiscal responsibility and accountability, regardless of the degree of delegation to others. Expenditures must be justifiable both in relation to the amounts allocated and in terms of the collection development policy.

The director must also assure that all those who carry out collection development responsibilities receive the appropriate training, ongoing guidance, and performance assessment. Because collection development encompasses a public relations role, the administrator must insure that staff with collection development responsibilities present a positive image of the library. Librarians who devote a significant proportion of time to collection development should have opportunities for professional growth, including continuing education and encouragement to undertake research or evaluative studies related to the collections.

The library director is also the ultimate spokesperson for the collections. It is the director to whom users will turn with complaints, and more rarely, compliments. The director will be called upon to address collection issues with faculty, institutional administrators, and affiliated organizations, such as Friends groups. For these reasons, even if not directly involved in collection development, the director must be fully aware of collection content, costs, and the policies that guide selection decisions and other collection development processes.

Job Descriptions

Each institution usually has a preferred format for job descriptions, but it is the content that is important. The Medical Library Association DocKit on *Position Descriptions in Health Sciences Libraries* contains job descriptions for many professional positions, but only two that encompass collection development responsibilities [12]. Listed below are some sample statements that have been drawn from a variety of collection development job descriptions.

- Manages selection activities in the library, including monographs, serials, audiovisuals, and computer software for all library locations.
- Plans and coordinates collection development policies.
- Makes recommendations for the annual collection budget.
- Monitors and documents publishing trends, interprets these trends to library staff and users, and assesses their budgetary impact.
- Assigns, supervises, and evaluates collection development activities of subject selectors.

- Selects materials in assigned subject areas, acting within the constraints of user needs, budget allocations, collection policies, and the library's strategic plan.

- Projects estimates and monitors expenditures of allocations for monographs and continuations.

- Exercises primary responsibility for planning and carrying out effective development of the library's collections in support of the university's teaching, research, patient care, and other programs.

- Establishes collection development policies and interprets them to staff, faculty, and others.

- Monitors gifts program; actively solicits gifts and coordinates and develops grant requests relating to collections.

- Reviews selection, deselection, replacement recommendations for large or unusual purchases, acceptance of large gifts, and conservation and storage policies in relation to the collection policy.

- Develops and oversees faculty liaison program with affiliated departments.

- Creates and maintains a central database of department profiles, including research profiles of individual faculty members.

- Develops and implements criteria and procedures for on-going evaluation of collections.

- Identifies needs to evaluate areas of the collection; guides or conducts evaluation studies.

- Reviews circulation reports and makes recommendations on purchase of additional copies and development of discrete subject collections.

- Monitors interlibrary loan reports to identify areas needing development and journal titles for which subscriptions should be entered.

- Uses knowledge of collections to improve and promote their use.

As is typical of job descriptions, these statements generally define the scope of responsibility or describe an activity but do not state the expected outcome of the responsibility. These statements can be modified to more truly reflect the goal rather than the process.

Description based: Assigns, supervises, and evaluates collection development activities of subject selectors.

Outcome based: Responsible for appropriate distribution of selection responsibilities, effective training and professional development programs for selectors, and collections that meet current user needs.

Description based: Develops and oversees faculty liaison program with affiliated departments.

Outcome based: Responsible for a faculty liaison program that results in active communication between the library and affiliated departments and informed advice on collections.

While these differences may seem trivial, the emphasis on outcomes more clearly defines a goal by which the program and the individual's performance may be measured.

Relationships within the Library

Collection Support Services

Collection development functions are intertwined with acquisition and bibliographic management activities. In some libraries collection development and acquisitions responsibilities are combined in a single position, reflecting their close relationship. While the activities and problems associated with obtaining materials (acquisitions) differ substantially from the activity of selecting and evaluating them, the processes interact. Purchase decisions must be transmitted from those who select to those who order or acquire. New subscription orders and cancellations should coincide with annual renewal cycles. Someone must make decisions about whether backfiles are desired. Preliminary searching may be undertaken by technical services staff, who pass on information regarding earlier editions of a text. Selectors may review materials received through approval plans. Those responsible for developing the collection may also provide advice on how a title should be handled bibliographically for easiest access (as a journal, analyzed, or cataloged separately) or on how it should be designated for circulation (noncirculating as a journal; loaned as a book).

While these interactions seem simple and obvious, if the mechanisms for communication are not in place and if the information—whether it flows from selectors to technical services staff, or vice versa—is neither expected nor encouraged, the communication path will be rocky or unreliable. Time will be wasted and valuable information lost. Relationships should be clearly defined and monitored to insure the best use of staff resources. (For further information on acquisitions, refer to Volume 5, *Acquisitions in Health Sciences Libraries.* For further information on cataloging, refer to Volume 6, *Bibliographic Management of Information Resources in Health Sciences Libraries.*)

Information Services

Because information services librarians interact with collection users on a daily basis, relationships with those providing direct client services are especially important to collection development. Even if they are not directly involved in collection development activities, input from these individuals is critical. When selectors are not also involved in user services, they must establish a link to those who are. If the library has designated one person for collection development, that individual should meet periodically with the information service librarians to discuss collection-related issues. If the library uses a group approach to decisions on journals, media, computer software, or electronic publications, public services staff should participate. If not, some mechanism for getting their recommendations is needed.

Systems Staff

As information sources in electronic formats become increasingly important components of local collections or are accessed through local systems, the library's systems experts and, in some cases staff outside the library, will need to be involved in these decisions. Decisions may involve issues of compatibility with local systems, functional capacity of equipment, a variety of operating platforms and protocols, and staffing needs for installation, maintenance, upgrading, and troubleshooting. Close working relationships with staff who have the appropriate technical knowledge are essential.

Borrowing and Document Delivery Services

Interlibrary loan and document procuring services are important adjuncts to collection development. Access is fast becoming integral to collection development as the dependence on external sources grows and local collections become more narrow. Copyright law demands that libraries either own materials or pay copyright charges when the fair use or CONTU guidelines are exceeded. Decisions regarding the cost-effectiveness of ownership over access become more complex as the speed and quality of document transmission improve and options for electronic access to full text increase. However, borrowing records continue to be important clues to local needs and those who select need to be alerted when the borrowing of specific titles reaches a predetermined threshold. Borrowing patterns by subject can point to new needs or weaknesses in the existing collection. They can also suggest areas where local ownership may not be needed. (For further information on copyright, refer to Volume 3, *Information Access and Delivery in Health Sciences Libraries.*)

Loan Services

Usage data are valuable in making selection decisions. Libraries with fully automated systems can easily get reports on the use of book collections, from general information, such as the relative use by subject classification, to very specific data, such as number of times an earlier edition of a text was used. Data on the number of holds placed on materials can be used to determine when multiple copies are needed. In-library use, especially for journals, media, and computer software, which in many libraries do not leave the library, can be measured by recording items reshelved, photocopy requests, computer accesses, or other means if not collected through the library's automated system. In libraries that are only partially automated or that rely on manual records, obtaining these types of data will depend more heavily on staff reporting. Circulation staff, especially when they are regular full-time staff, can be valuable sources of information about use patterns and current demands for materials. Decisions about replacing lost books are collection development decisions, but they also depend on a smooth flow of information from circulation to collection development and then on to acquisitions or bibliographic control staff. Libraries will have different pathways; what is critical is to clearly delineate the path.

Relationships with Users

While usage data from library records and knowledge of needs from library staff play an essential part in deciding what to purchase, they do not substitute for direct contact with library users. User contact can be established in numerous ways.

Library Committees

Most libraries, regardless of the institutional setting, have a library committee, board, or advisory group of some type. These bodies may perform a variety of roles with respect to the collections, from approving the library's budget, to advising on the collection's scope and purpose, to approving individual journal or even book purchases. Although the size of the institution will partially dictate the degree to which an advisory body may become involved, in most cases the library will want to have control over individual purchase decisions. A library committee should know and endorse the stated purpose of the library and the scope of its collections as defined in a written policy. The library then has an approved framework in which to make decisions but retains the flexibility to determine what materials will best meet institutional needs. With stagnant or shrinking budgets, an advisory committee may provide support for seeking additional funding or to back the library's actions when unpopular journal cancellations become necessary. If involved in advance, they may not only assist in planning an approach to budget reductions, but communicate with their colleagues in ways that the librarian cannot.

Institutional Administration

Whenever possible, the library should seek ways to participate within the administrative structure of the institution. This participation can be accomplished in several ways, depending on the nature and complexity of the institution. The library director or other librarians may find opportunities for involvement in functions, such as:

- Senior management group.
- Department or service heads group.
- Planning committees.
- Continuing education or in-service training committees.
- Curriculum-related committees.
- Quality assurance leadership groups.
- Facilitator for total quality management (TQM) or similar programs.
- Historical committee.
- Accreditation self-study group.

Information gained from participation in groups such as these can be invaluable in determining the direction of the institution and assessing how the library can best support its users. It can have direct implications for collection development.

Department Liaisons

Retaining autonomy over collection decisions does not mean a library should make those decisions without some method of getting direct input from users. A small hospital or clinic library with a very specialized group of users and a very limited budget will rely more heavily on advice from its clientele than will a large academic health sciences library serving multiple professional schools and a broad range of research and training programs. Even the largest library, however, needs to consult with its clientele; indeed, as budgets get tighter and the selection process more precise, user input in large libraries becomes critical to collection development decisions. A liaison program with representatives from the different schools and departments served by the library encourages communication between faculty and library and conveys the message that the library listens to its users. Faculty consultants can evaluate new journals, gathering opinions from others in their departments. They can assist with reviewing current subscriptions for cancellation or assessing the library's coverage of their discipline, or advise on the needed depth of collecting to support departmental research programs.

If the library either invites volunteers or asks department heads to appoint a liaison to the library, it is wise to 1) describe the characteristics desired of a representative and 2) acknowledge that the faculty member's time is valuable and demands on it will be made judiciously and sparingly. While it is a common practice to assign younger faculty to library committees, this can have disadvantages: they may have less cumulative knowledge of the field (journals, publishers, editors, authors), and if they are not yet tenured, may be under greater time pressures for research, grant writing, publishing, and teaching. A senior member of the faculty may be a better choice for this role. The library needs to make clear that a consultant should be someone who knows the field, is able to represent fairly department-wide needs (not just their own), will consult with others, and is willing to respond when advice is needed. In turn, the library should minimize the time required of the faculty and use them wisely. In times of major changes, such as large-scale journal cancellations, all faculty may need to be involved, but the consultants can play a coordinating role.

The librarians, especially those who serve as selectors in the corresponding subject areas, should maintain contact with the department consultants. They can do this by attending lectures, seminars, or other events and by making sure the consultants are kept informed about developments in the library. To complement a faculty liaison program or simply to establish direct links to user groups, the library may also designate individual librarians as liaisons to specific departments or services. The library should consider establishing links with specialized groups, such as patient education, dietetics, laboratory animal care, and administration, as well as academic departments, research institutes, and clinical services. The librarian liaisons serve as a communication channel regarding the collection; they often act more broadly to communicate with user groups on other library services, such as education programs or electronic resources. Liaison programs are an effective method to increase the library's visibility and maintain positive library-user relationships.

Suggestions from Users

In addition to advisory bodies and formalized liaison plans, the library needs methods for conveying information to its users about the collections and for gathering comments and specific suggestions. Suggestion boxes and forms for recommending books and journals are common methods of soliciting recommendations. Request forms may be a choice through the library's electronic catalog or communications network, or the library may receive recommendations through electronic mail from its users. Newsletter articles (institutional as well as library), bulletin boards, exhibits, and new book displays can promote the collections by highlighting new or specialized materials. Graphic capabilities on electronic information servers offer a variety of possibilities for increasing awareness of collection resources.

Institutional Relationships

Library consortia and resource sharing agreements are discussed in detail in Chapter 10, Cooperative Collection Development. In an academic environment, the relationships between the health sciences libraries and the general academic library are important. They are mandated if the health sciences library is part of a university library system. In a multilibrary system, coordination with other science branch libraries will be needed. Because of interdisciplinary needs, the health sciences library will also need to interact with those responsible for collections in the social sciences and disciplines such as health care administration, architecture, social work, and education.

In hospitals or other clinical settings, patient or health education libraries may be separate from the health sciences library. If so, some effort may be required to share information and coordinate collections. Drug information centers and health sciences libraries can have a mutually beneficial relationship in developing collections and providing access to specialized drug resources. As integrated systems in medical centers begin to tie together patient records and other information resources, libraries and medical records departments also need to work more closely together. Those responsible for collections and knowledgeable about their use need to be involved in decisions about which resources are made available through the institutional information system and how to link them to local patient information. In a corporate pharmaceutical setting, technical or research libraries may be separate from more clinically related collections, requiring some mechanism for sharing information and coordinating collections.

Relationships with Publishers, Vendors, and Authors

Less obvious, but equally critical to library collections, are the roles played by the publishers, vendors, and authors.

Publishers

Publishers decide the format for disseminating information: single book, series, journal, supplement, loose-leaf, CD-ROM, or floppy disk. They determine frequency for journals, new editions, and updates. Each of these publisher decisions results in a corresponding library decision: whether to place a standing order for a series or only get selected volumes; whether a new edition of a text or reference book is needed; whether to get paper copy if an electronic version is available. Publishers act as selectors when libraries establish continuation orders, blanket order plans, and depository agreements, because the library acquires everything within the agreed-upon scope issued by the publisher, whether a government agency, professional association, or commercial publisher. Surprisingly little interaction between publishers and librarians takes place regarding the decisions made by publishers, even for reference works. However, some biomedical publishers do include librarians on their advisory committees or have established advisory groups comprised entirely of collection development librarians. Such groups play an important communications role between the producer and the ultimate distributor of that information. This practice should be encouraged, with librarians taking a more active role as an advocate for their own needs and those of their users.

Vendors

The vendor, in the middle between the publisher and the library purchaser, has an important relationship to collection development functions, frequently through the acquisitions process. The speed with which a vendor supplies an order, for example, directly affects how soon an item is added to the collection. In managing an approval plan, the vendor acts as a surrogate selector—deciding what fits a library's profile and what does not. An approval plan needs to be carefully crafted and followed up with regular monitoring and communication by both parties to assure that it continues to meet the library's needs. Cumulative data on publishing and pricing trends specific to the library provided by vendors are used in making budget and selection decisions. Librarians should work closely with vendors, understanding that the vendor functions with two sets of restraints—those imposed by the publishers and those imposed by the library customers. Library needs will more likely be met if librarians maintain active communication.

Relationships with vendors raise many of the same issues for collection development librarians as they do for librarians involved with serials management and acquisitions. Librarians should work as colleagues with vendors; they have many concerns in common, such as knowledge about what is being published, current costs and future projections, and criteria by which libraries select materials. Collaboration is necessary if vendors are to tailor services to meet actual needs. Librarians must also be sensitive to such matters as conflict of interest, acceptance of gifts or travel expenses, and other benefits. What may appear to be part of normal business dealings to a vendor may not be acceptable within an institution's guidelines, especially a state institution, or may raise ethical questions. It is essential for librarians to know and understand their institution's requirements with regard to interactions with vendors or outside organizations.

Authors

Most often missing in the collection development process is the link between the librarian and the author or creator of a work. Librarians responsible for collection development decisions know a lot about what information is used and what is not used. They constantly measure cost against value. They may complain about what gets published and the demands placed on the library to purchase materials that do not meet needs well, whether it is yet another slim but high priced immunology journal or a CD-ROM index that has a cumbersome interface and is updated only once a year. Librarians should assume the frequently neglected role as an advocate for the consumer—not only the library as consumer, but the physician or student or researcher as consumer. Much of the work that gets published comes from the libraries' own institutions or is sponsored by professional societies to which their users belong. They have strong and potentially influential links to the authors of biomedical literature, but too often librarians fail to take advantage of opportunities to communicate collection issues effectively to authors. This role as advocate needs strengthening.

References

1. Bryant B. The organizational structure of collection development. Libr Res Tech Serv 1987 Apr-Jun; 31(2):111-122.

2. Cogswell J. The organization of collection management functions in academic research libraries. J Acad Libr 1987 Nov; 13(5):268-276.

3. Pitschmann LA. Organization and staffing. In: Osborn CB, Atkinson R, eds. Collection management: a new treatise. Greenwich, CT: JAI Press, 1991:125-143. (Foundations in library and information science, v. 26).

4. Sohn J. Collection development organizational patterns in ARL libraries. Libr Res Tech Serv. 1987 Apr-Jun; 31(2):123-134.

5. Dudley NH. Organizational models for collection development. In: Stueart RD, ed. Collection development in libraries: a treatise. Greenwich, CT: JAI Press, 1980. (Foundations in library and information science, v.10).

6. Collection development organization and staffing in ARL libraries. Washington, DC: Association of Research Libraries, 1987. (SPEC Kit no. 131).

7. Creth SD. The organization of collection development: a shift in the organization paradigm. J Libr Admin 1991; 14(1):67-85.

8. Law D. The organization of collection management in academic libraries. In: Jenkins C, Morley M, eds. Collection management in academic libraries. Aldershot, England: Gower, 1991:3.

9. Morse D. Staffing patterns in collection development and acquisitions. Biomed Libr Acq Bull [serial online] 1993 Oct 22; no. 22:1.7. Available from: University of Southern California, Norris Medical Library, Los Angeles via Internet.

10. Robinson WC. Academic library collection development and management positions: announcements in College and Research Libraries News from 1980 through 1991. Libr Res Tech Serv 1993 Apr; 37(2):134-146.

11. Staffing patterns in collection development and acquisitions. Biomed Lib Acq Bull. [serial online] 1993 Oct 18, no. 20; Oct 19, no. 21; Oct 22, no. 22. Available from: University of Southern California, Norris Medical Library, Los Angeles via Internet.

12. Weaver CG, comp. Position descriptions in health sciences libraries. Chicago: Medical Library Association, 1989. (MLA DocKit no. 1).

3

Education and Training for Collection Development

"It's all to do with training: you can do a lot if you're properly trained."
Elizabeth II,
Queen of Great Britain and
Northern Ireland

Collection development is multi-faceted and encompasses a variety of functions. This chapter examines the factors most likely to lead to success in this subfield of librarianship. It looks at what characteristics are important and what knowledge is essential for those who have responsibility for one or more aspects of collection development in health sciences libraries. It suggests where and how they can acquire the necessary knowledge and skills for success in this area of professional specialization.

Knowledge and Skills

Each aspect of collection development demands somewhat different skills. Four broad functions are examined: selector, evaluator, coordinator, and administrator.

The Selector

Selectors make the basic decisions: they determine that the library should subscribe to a new specialty journal; they choose which anatomical atlas to acquire; they weigh the advantages of an electronic version over paper copy; they decide whether a new edition of a textbook is needed; they assess the need for the printed proceedings of a conference. These are the practical decisions regarding which materials are acquired by the library and which are not. While selectors do not always make these decisions alone, and in the case of very expensive or long-term commitments, rarely do, they play a key role. Whether making decisions from publishers' announcements, reviewing books received through approval plans, or responding to user requests, the expertise needed by selectors is similar.

Subject Knowledge

Bibliographers in large academic libraries frequently have advanced degrees in the subjects for which they are responsible. This is uncommon in health sciences libraries. Few health sciences libraries are so large that they have more than one librarian solely, or even mostly, devoted to collection development responsibilities. While librarians with degrees in nursing, public health, and biological sciences are not rare, an M.D. librarian is extremely unusual. The library that is able to hire librarians with subject backgrounds in the biological or health sciences in addition to other required abilities is fortunate. Whatever their formal training, however, selectors need to understand the subject field(s) being selected. Selectors need the following skills:

- Familiarity with the specialized terminology.
- Understanding of basic concepts and importance of the field.
- Awareness of current controversies.
- Recognition of names of prominent researchers.
- Knowledge of historical milestones and the names associated with them.
- Understanding of how the field relates to other health science disciplines.

Knowledge of the Publishing World

Selectors need to know about publishers and the publishing process. They need to understand the steps involved in publishing books, journals, and electronic resources, and the factors a publisher considers in making decisions. Selectors need to know what types of materials major medical publishers specialize in, the quality of materials they put out, their reliability, their pricing practices, and their general reputation, both in the publishing world and the library world. Collection development librarians need to maintain an awareness of publishing trends, production statistics, prices, and other industry indications.

Selectors need to understand the role of vendors and how they relate to the publishing and distribution process and what effect their participation has on collection development routines. Vendors often employ librarians as representatives; these individuals can play an important collegial role with collection librarians.

Selectors should not only be familiar with what has been published in the health sciences, but they need to know the standard texts and primary clinical and research journals within each major discipline. They need to know the important series and reference works, the most authoritative and comprehensive electronic files and databases.

The confusing and changing world of intellectual property rights, copyright law, and licensing agreements poses a challenge to those making resource management decisions. These are thorny issues, open to various interpretations and legal challenges, and it is important for selectors to be knowledgeable about them.

Critical Judgment

A selector must be able to analyze information and make decisions. Technology and economic restraints have transformed the world in which libraries function. The environment in which selections are made forces the selector to consider such factors as choices between various formats or media, alternative forms of access, and associated equipment and staff costs. As a result, selection can be difficult. The range of criteria to be weighed is wider now than it used to be, making the process more complex. The selector needs not only the knowledge on which to base decisions, but the ability to weigh alternatives and take action based on critical analysis of the choices. Criteria by which to judge the quality of a publication—both the content and its packaging—must be established and the selector must be able to apply these criteria and to assess benefits in relation to costs.

Knowledge of User Needs

Users' requirements for information resources, whether journals, media, books, or electronic files, should be anticipated by the selector—not every title, of course, but the library must do more than simply respond to user demands. Selectors should know their institution: research interests, the case mix of the hospital, residency and fellowship programs, large-scale training grants, required and recommended texts for students.

Knowledge of Technology

Medical information is transmitted through a growing array of technologies. Paper is now only one of several media acquired by libraries. As more resources are available in electronic formats, whether as CD-ROMs, interactive video disks, or hypertext programs, the collection development librarian must be aware of the special characteristics, benefits and disadvantages of each. Electronic resources may be on single workstations or local area networks within the library, mounted on institutional networks, or accessed through global networks like the Internet. For each type of application the selector will need to be familiar with the structure, characteristics, and technical requirements.

Not only must they be familiar with the electronic formats, but selectors should also have skills in navigating these resources and be able to evaluate them in terms of access, ease of use, and manipulability. They need to have a basic knowledge of hardware requirements, networking, and communications software.

The Evaluator

Evaluation and selection go hand in hand. Initial selection of materials is an evaluative function, as it is a judgment of value of an individual item in relation to the collection as a whole. However, evaluation of collections considers a universe of materials. Collection evaluation requires special skills beyond those needed for ongoing selection of new materials.

Subject Knowledge

Considerable knowledge of a discipline is essential to conduct a thorough evaluation of how well the library is covering that field and how well it meets the needs of that segment of the library's clientele. While use of consulting subject specialists is common and usually valuable, the librarian evaluator should be more than superficially familiar with the subject area. The evaluator must know enough to select an appropriate method for evaluation and must be able to recognize definitive works, sources that can be used for benchmarks, and the location of special collections which supplement local holdings or with which to compare local holdings.

Knowledge of User Needs

Collection evaluation doesn't take place in isolation from the library's purpose. The collection must always be evaluated in relation to *something*. In most health science libraries that *something* is the needs of the primary user population. For this reason, the evaluator must understand the library's clientele and the specific demands it has for information. It makes a difference whether the library serves high profile, intense research programs, whether the institution has established centers of excellence in specific clinical or research areas, or has specialized training programs with unique information requirements. The evaluator must know the context in which the collections have been developed and are used.

Research Skills

An evaluator needs to be familiar with different techniques for gathering data and analyzing results. The choice of an appropriate and practical method can make the difference between useful information acquired in a cost-effective manner or considerable time and effort spent on unreliable results. Although the techniques will differ, research skills are also needed to conduct a valid assessment of information needs. In addition to general familiarity with research methods, the evaluator should have a good understanding of the various methods used to evaluate collections, including collection-based and client-based approaches. The ability to interpret data and draw conclusions from them complements the ability to select and apply methods, and is equally important. The evaluator needs an analytical mind to make sense out of gathered information and to formulate recommendations based on that information.

The Coordinator

In libraries with several librarians who have responsibilities for collection development, one person will have overall responsibility. Whether this position assumes a supervisory role or only a coordinating role, similar characteristics are important. Even if collection development is centralized in a single person rather than being shared among several librarians, a coordinating function is embedded in the responsibility. To the skills of a selector and evaluator, the coordinator must add interpersonal, teaching, and supervisory skills.

Interpersonal Skills

The stereotype of the academic bibliographer is one who concentrates on an ultraspecialized esoteric field. The selector with the green eye-shade does not apply in health sciences libraries and has largely disappeared from academic libraries. The coordinator, in particular, must interpret policy, allocate scarce resources among competing needs, negotiate shared or divided responsibilities among libraries on a campus or in a consortium, and deal with faculty or health professionals who are unhappy when materials important to them are not acquired. These responsibilities demand objectivity, sensitivity to multiple and not necessarily compatible needs, and the ability to work cooperatively with others.

Teaching Skills

The coordinator is often also the educator, responsible for the training and continuing education of selectors and evaluators. The coordinator should be expected to develop training plans, identify needs for expanding subject knowledge or research skills, and carry out an effective educational program, either formally or informally. This skill is an all too frequently neglected component in collection development; teaching skills are not often considered requirements for such positions.

Supervisory Skills

Direct supervision may or may not be a function of the coordinator, however, the traits of a good supervisor—working with individuals to set goals, establishing standards for performance, providing coaching to solve problems, and evaluating results—are valuable whether the relationship is direct or indirect.

The Administrator

Depending on the library, the collection administrator may not be a selector, evaluator, or coordinator, or may have all or some of these functions. The administrator recommends or establishes policy, participates in setting performance standards for those involved in collection development, and prepares and manages collection budgets.

Financial Analysis

The administrator should be able to apply effective techniques for cost analysis and projections and to interpret financial data on cost of collection materials. This person should know the sources of information about projected prices, economic trends, and changes in scientific publishing. An understanding of the economics of information is also important for the administrator. Knowledge of the local institutional budget structure, financial conditions, and fiscal practices are essential.

Policy Formation

In most cases, the library director will have ultimate responsibility for the collections, as well as for all other library functions. It is the director, usually in consultation with an advisory body and institutional administrators, who establishes and oversees the broad guiding policies for the collections, the principles on which collection activities are based. Because it is the director who must assure that the library's collection policies complement and support institutional goals, this person must clearly understand the institution and the direction it is taking. In establishing, interpreting, and sometimes defending policies to users, the library administrator must also exercise negotiating skills and diplomacy.

Administrative Skills

Management abilities expected of any library administrator should be applied to collection development activities. In libraries where collection development functions are divided among several staff and do not comprise a majority of any single person's job, management functions such as planning, aside from budget considerations; performance standards; staff development; and evaluation may tend to be neglected.

Having described four different roles as if they were separate persons or distinct positions, it should be pointed out that these distinctions are very unlikely to exist in pure form in any health sciences library. The chief librarian in a one- or two-librarian situation will encompass all roles. In a large academic health sciences library, these functions may be concentrated in different positions, but with some of each function in more than one position. Furthermore, the depth of knowledge required for each of these roles will also vary considerably depending on the size and nature of the library, its budget, and the institution it serves. The roles have been described separately to illustrate specialized skills required for different functions.

Preprofessional Preparation and Graduate Education

Undergraduate Background

Except for those few who have made a career change to librarianship from one of the health-related professions, subject knowledge in the life sciences is most likely to be acquired during undergraduate education. Knowledge in the biological or health sciences is especially valuable for collection development responsibilities. Academic preparation in any of the sciences should also provide students with a good understanding of the scientific process, a grounding in analytical techniques, and exposure to the scientific literature.

Graduate Library Education

Can collection development be taught or is it an art for which some have the aptitude and others do not? Even if there is an element of "art" in selecting materials—serendipity, a sensitivity to users, the ability to anticipate needs—there must be a solid foundation of knowledge and understanding. Knowledge drawn from a number of disciplines contributes greatly to success in building and managing collections. Librarians need to know about the sociology of science and scientific communication, the process by which new medical knowledge is diffused. Librarians should understand the medical community they serve—what information physicians or other health professionals need and how they go about getting it. They should understand and be able to apply principles of information science to establishing collection policies and developing collections.

Graduate education in library and information science has been reexamined in the 1990s: some library schools have been closed, new alliances are being forged with other academic disciplines, and the educational needs of the modern information professional are being evaluated. Among the competencies that Woodsworth and Lester have suggested graduates will need to meet library needs in the 21st century are several with direct implications for collection development and management:

"Understanding of the characteristics of information transfer, including users' information seeking behavior and information-generating activities within the various disciplines."

"Skill in identifying and analyzing the information needs of various constituencies served and how these information needs could be met through the complex of information agencies."

"Skill in evaluating information and a willingness to make relevant decisions based on expertise in both information management and subject areas of disciplines."

"Understanding of and ability to analyze information policy issues, including legal issues...and regulatory issues and structures...."

"Understanding of the impact of both the national and international economy on information access, e.g., the effects produced by the costs of resources, trade restrictions, inflation, and changes in the tax structure."

"Understanding of the generation, production, and distribution of information and of the changing paradigm as shifts occur from print-based information production to other modes of production and dissemination" [1].

Graduate programs vary in content from school to school. Metz, who surveyed the course offerings in a group of highly rated library schools, found a small majority required a course on collection development or collection development and acquisitions. Most others incorporated collection development topics in other required courses [2]. A broader survey found that reference and cataloging were the only consistently required courses [3]. General courses in collection development may touch on specialized collections but do not deal specifically with the health sciences; health sciences library courses rarely devote more than perhaps a lecture or two on collections. Both the theoretical issues related to collection policy, assessment, and organization, and the practical applications such as selection and budget management are treated superficially or not at all. While courses in research methods are taught and often required, collection assessment techniques may not be included. Graduates of library education programs should have a thorough grounding in evaluation techniques and understand how to take advantage of automated systems for collection analysis, cost trends, cost and benefit determination, and collection-use studies. Not all programs fulfill this need. Johnson has suggested that preparation for collection development responsibilities include grounding in financial skills, statistical skills, organizational behavior, ethical considerations, communication skills, marketing and fund raising, and decision making [4].

Graduate Education in Specialized Disciplines

Librarians who have entered the field from nursing, medical technology, public health, pharmacy, dietetics, or other health careers often bring with them not only a subject background and familiarity with medical terminology, but a broad understanding of practice-based information needs. This understanding complements the more common research-based focus of librarians who come from academic environments. Few librarians seriously pursue professional training in health fields for the purpose of improving their contributions to librarianship. At mid-career, the financial burden and lost time are significant and difficult to justify, as direct rewards for additional training are unlikely. Graduate education in basic sciences such as molecular biology, nutrition, public health, or biochemistry is more common. Whether these advanced degrees precede or follow entry into health sciences librarianship, the knowledge acquired can often be applied directly to collection development activity by improving the ability to exercise critical judgment, assess content quality, and place individual publications within the context of the entire literature of the field. Advanced degrees in the sciences also add to the credibility of selectors as they work with faculty or physicians. Expertise in the sciences, however, does not guarantee an effective selector or evaluator and may even be a source of friction with a coordinator or administrator. A librarian planning to work with rare books or special collections may need more intense education in history of science and medicine, archival techniques, or discipline-specific knowledge.

On-the-Job Training

Even when the fundamentals of collection development have been taught in graduate school and the student has been exposed to a range of biomedical and health literature, the new graduate librarian is ill-equipped to take on collection development responsibilities. According to Creth, "the primary objective of job training is to bring about a change—an increase in knowledge, the acquisition of a skill, or the development of confidence and good judgment" [5]. All three functions have a place in collection development training.

There are two approaches to on-the-job training: the sink-or-swim approach and the systematic approach. In the worst, and all too frequent, case of sink-or-swim, the librarian is given subject areas to cover, or in a small library maybe all selection responsibilities, and told the procedures for forwarding items to be ordered. Maybe the person has a budget within which to operate. Maybe someone else, a collection development librarian or the director or even a committee, reviews final selections and maybe that person or group gives the selector some comments or suggestions. Although the librarian may eventually (and if alert and ambitious, probably will) learn to do the job well, this approach should not be considered adequate training.

Systematic Training and Guided Experience

There is no substitute for education through apprenticeship when the teacher is an expert and is willing to share that knowledge by working directly with the learner. With a master teacher the novice learns by observation, by listening, and finally by doing. However, in most situations time and staffing limitations dictate a more structured experience. The American Library Association (ALA) has recommended content for a practical collection development handbook which may be helpful to those responsible for training new collection development staff [6]. Before starting a training program the instructor should establish objectives—what is expected of the individual at the end of the program. Training for collection development might include some of the following objectives. At the conclusion of training the new selector:

- Knows how the institution is organized and understands the scope and emphasis of its programs.

- Is familiar with the breadth and depth of the existing library collections, including any special collections, their strengths and weaknesses, and the history of their development.

- Knows the library's policies and guidelines related to the collections, including those for special formats and various audience levels, as well as subject scope.

- Understands the library's budget for collections; is familiar with how it is allocated and administered.

- Knows about any cooperative agreements or arrangements for shared information with other libraries on campus, in a consortium, or in the region.

- Understands the basic content of copyright law as it pertains to libraries, and guidelines for applying the law.
- Is familiar with the standard works in the disciplines covered and with benchmark bibliographies, core lists, and other reference sources.
- Is familiar with the characteristics of major scientific journal and book publishers.
- Uses multiple sources for information about new books, journals, and other media. Knows how to find authoritative reviews when needed.
- Knows the library's staff and other individuals in the institution who can contribute to or be called upon in carrying out collection development routines and functions.
- Can apply collection policies and selection criteria to choosing new materials for the library.
- Can conduct an objective and valid review of a subject area, applying appropriate research methods.

As it is unlikely that more than one or two librarians will be undergoing training at any one time, the program can be tailored to individual needs, eliminating those aspects already familiar to the individual. For example, when training someone who has already been in the library for several years but in another job, information about the institution may not be needed. A recent graduate who has taken a comprehensive medical libraries course should be familiar with core lists.

The size of the library and its organization for collection development will determine who conducts the training. Most often it will be the person who has overall responsibility for collection development. The methods by which each objective is to be achieved should be outlined and time scheduled for it. Some suggestions follow.

Reading

- Materials related to the medical school, hospital, or other local health programs such as catalogs, brochures on residencies or training programs, annual reports, planning documents, descriptions of recently awarded grants, faculty publication lists.
- Collection policy for the library and for other campus or affiliated libraries.

- Profile of the library's approval plan, if it has one.

- Bryant B, ed. *Guide for Written Collection Policy Statements.* Chicago: American Library Association, 1989 (Collection management and collection guides, no. 3).

- Morse DH, Richards DT, comp. *Collection Development Policies for Health Sciences Libraries.* Chicago: Medical Library Association, 1992. (MLA DocKit no. 3).

- Introductions to the most recent editions of the Brandon/Hill lists.

- Richards DT. *Development and Assessment of Health Sciences Library Collections.* Chicago: Medical Library Association, 1992. (MLA CE701).

- Selected articles related to various aspects of book and journal publishing: structured abstracts, peer review, pricing practices, electronic publishing, copyright.

Examples:

Structured abstracts

- Haynes RB, Mulrow CD, Huth EJ, Altman DG, Gardner MJ. More informative abstracts revisited. *Ann Intern Med* 1990 Jul 1; 113(1):69-76.

- Mulrow CD, Thaker SP, Pugh JA. A proposal for more informative abstracts of review articles. *Ann Intern Med* 1988 Apr; 108(4):613-5.

- A proposal for more informative abstracts of clinical articles. Ad Hoc Working Group for Critical Appraisal of the Medical Literature. *Ann Intern Med* 1987 Apr; 106(4):598-604.

Peer review

- Lock S. *A Difficult Balance: Editorial Peer Review in Medicine.* Philadelphia: ISI Press, 1986.

- *Peer Review in Scientific Publishing.* Chicago: Council of Biology Editors, 1991.

- Second International Congress on Peer Review in Biomedical Publication. *JAMA* 1994 Jul 13; 272(2):91-173.

Pricing

- *Newsletter on Serials Pricing Issues* [serial online]. Available from Office of Information Technology, Univ. North Carolina at Chapel Hill via INTERNET - LISTSERV@UNC.EDU.

- Serial vendor newsletters and periodic reports.
- *Library Issues: Briefings for Faculty and Administrators.* Ann Arbor, MI: Mountainside Publishing. Contains frequent articles relating to journal cost issues, written for nonlibrarian audience.

Copyright

- Matheson N. Copyrights and the user's rights: an editorial. *Bull Med Libr Assoc* 1993 Jul; 81(3):330-1.
- Bennett S, Matheson N. Scholarly articles: valuable commodities for universities. *Chron Higher Educ* 1992 May 27; 1-3.
- *The Copyright Law and the Health Science Librarian.* Chicago: Medical Library Association, 1989.

Materials to Examine

- Current journals subscribed to by the library.
- Book collection.
- Reference collection.
- Reserve collection.
- Electronic resources and other media.
- Special collections.
- Publishers' catalogs and announcements.
- Library journals specializing in collection development:
  - *Biomedical Library Acquisitions Bulletin* (BLAB) [serial online]. Univ. Southern California, Norris Medical Library, Los Angeles, CA.
  - *Collection Building* (New York: Neal-Schuman).
  - *Collection Management* (Binghamton, NY: Haworth Press).
  - *Library Acquisitions: Practice & Theory* (Elmsford, NY: Pergamon Press).
  - *Library Journal* (New York: Cahners Publishing Co.).
  - *Publishers Weekly* (New York: Cahners Publishing Co.).
  - *Serials Review* (Greenwich, CT: JAI Press).
- Information sources within the library: search requests, ILL data, reference question information such as forms, files, computer-based data collection and reports.

- Book reviews in science and medical journals that may be used for selection and general knowledge of new developments in the health sciences: *Academic Medicine, American Journal of Nursing, JAMA, New England Journal of Medicine, Nature, Science.*

Discussion Topics

- Collection policies and how they are applied.
- Criteria for selecting journals, books, software, media.
- Selected issues raised from readings.
- Procedures including flow of information and work.

Practice and Review

- Select materials of various types.
- Review criteria used in making decisions.
- Choose a subject area and conduct a preliminary evaluation.
- Review methods and results.

Contacts to Make

- Other selectors.
- Staff who provide user service in reference, interlibrary loan, and circulation.
- Technical services staff: review approval plans, gifts, standing orders, deposit plans, exchange plans, data available through the automated library system.
- Faculty liaisons or other groups of library users, library committee members.
- Other librarians in the institution, especially those who select in related subjects.
- Other health science librarians in the region. Visit libraries where there is interaction as part of a consortium or other cooperative programs.
- Publisher and vendor representatives with whom the library does significant business.

Additional suggestions may be found in the sample training programs published by the Association of Research Libraries (ARL) [7].

Self-Directed Learning

Even if no organized training is offered, an individual who has taken on selection or collection development responsibilities can still benefit from a systematic learning process. After identifying the goals of a self-directed training plan, the person should identify the resources (documents, readings, people) needed and set aside time to follow through. This process will require considerably more discipline than a library-directed training process, but will allow the person to gain knowledge and competence more quickly than simply picking up information over time.

Those who take on collection responsibilities for unfamiliar disciplines must take steps to acquire subject knowledge. Selectors with a nonscience background will find it useful to undertake some reading about the scientific method. Within subject areas familiarity and recognition are more important than detailed knowledge. Knowing the science is not essential; knowing the important concepts, issues, and people is.

Reading histories or biographies will help a selector recognize names and some of the many diseases, syndromes, techniques or instruments named after those who first described or developed them. Reading the introductions to new books and rationale statements in new journals, scanning general textbooks, annual reviews and symposium proceedings will provide good background and an overview of subjects within the library's scope. Familiarity with current scientific advances and important names can be gained by regular review of general science journals, such as *Science, Nature, New Scientist,* and the essays in *Current Contents.* Both *JAMA* and *New England Journal of Medicine* are good sources to keep up with current issues in clinical medicine. The "Contempo" issue of *JAMA*, published annually since 1978, contains short summaries of developments in many areas of medicine [8]. Primary care and selected other specialties are covered annually, other topics biennially or reviewed every three to five years. It may help new selectors to make lists of prominent journal editors, biomedical prize winners, officers in major medical societies, and other leaders. Attending lectures, seminars, and grand rounds, and when feasible, departmental faculty meetings will provide insight into local research and patient care interests. For special interests the selector may audit relevant courses.

Continuing Education

Formal Education

Workshops and continuing education courses are sponsored by the Medical Library Association (MLA), ARL, other library associations, graduate library schools, and even vendors. Those attending vendor courses should always be aware of potential bias if the content focuses on proprietary products or vendor-specific services. Often a seminar or workshop may focus on some aspect of collection development, such as serials or collection evaluation. The Association for Library Collections and Technical Services (ALCTS) has for many years conducted a series of collection management and development institutes, which offer opportunities for librarians to learn the basics of collection management theories and practice. A series of advanced institutes facilitates the exploration of trends and changes in the collection development specialty. Attending continuing education programs outside the institution offers the benefit of interaction with individuals from a variety of institutions, resulting in new insights, ideas, and techniques, as well as a greater understanding of issues. Participants usually identify colleagues with whom they can consult in the future.

Informal Education

Librarians have a proclivity to organize around special interests; collection development librarians are no exception. One of the formal sections within the MLA is devoted to collection development. At a broader level, the Charleston (SC) Annual Conference focuses on issues in acquisitions and collection development. Specialized organizations, such as the North American Serials Interest Group (NASIG), draw together people with common concerns.

At a local level, regional chapters of MLA or other library groups may provide opportunities to meet with other collection development librarians, to share problems and solutions, and in the process contribute to continuing education.

Electronic communications, including e-mail, listservs, bulletin boards and conferencing software, offer numerous opportunities to share information, ideas, and expertise with colleagues. Special interest groups on the Internet emerge and fade as issues wax and wane. Electronic networks provide access to reports, data, and documents. Interactive discussions take place on issues such as journal pricing, mergers of publishers and vendors, copyright, electronic publishing, and software licensing.

Performance Appraisal

Librarians with collection development or management responsibilities should have the benefit of guidance and constructive evaluation. Frequently, where collection activities are distributed among staff who have reference, teaching, or technical service responsibilities as well, these other functions are viewed as the primary role and are the focus of performance evaluation by department heads or other supervisors. The collection development function may be neglected. This may be especially true if the collection coordinator does not have a clear management role. When the organizational hierarchy prevalent in libraries is mixed with a more lateral or matrix approach to collection responsibilities, performance review for collection development tends to be abandoned.

Responsibility for Assessment

If collections constitute an important element of library service—and for the foreseeable future they probably will continue to do so—then evaluating the work of those responsible for those collections is also important. Goal-setting and performance appraisal for collection development should be included in the library's regular cycle of planning and review. Who conducts the reviews will be determined by the size and organization of the library. If leadership for collection development is outside the normal reporting structure, then supplementary reviews from the collection coordinator or peers may be obtained by the supervisor.

Job Description and Goals

Developing effective criteria for reviewing performance related to collection development can be a challenge. The starting point should be the individual's job description. The percent of time expected to be devoted to collection activities will be a guide to how much the individual should reasonably be expected to accomplish. Specific expectations with respect to collection evaluation, consultation with faculty, and budget management should be clear. In addition to ongoing responsibilities, goals established each year and amended or added to throughout the year should be referred to in any assessment of work accomplished. Examples might include

- Assess nursing collection.
- Develop criteria for preservation.

- Conduct needs assessment in biotechnology.
- Create journal evaluation database.

Measuring the Process

A focus on process is at least two steps removed from truly measuring effectiveness in collection development. It is nevertheless useful as one indicator of performance and it is far easier to measure. Are books selected and orders forwarded on a timely basis; are the statistics collected thorough and accurate; are approval books or new books evaluated according to established routines in a timely fashion; is a broad array of sources used for selection; are requests from users handled promptly; does the individual pursue continuing education opportunities; is communication with others in the process positive and helpful? If the individual has fund management responsibilities, is spending controlled; are reports prompt and informative? Are preservation responsibilities undertaken actively; are weeding or assessment projects carried out according to plans; are faculty or other users consulted regularly? These questions address how efficiently individuals use time, how well they adhere to routines, and how well they work with others, and are therefore important to the library, but can only be used in conjunction with other measures.

Measuring Knowledge

Knowledge of the collection, knowledge of the subject, and knowledge of the users are all essential ingredients to effective collection development. These attributes are more difficult to measure than process and depend more on indirect indicators and subjective opinion. Is the person sought out by users for information regarding the collection and turned to for advice by colleagues? Does the individual contribute knowledgeably to discussions, give evidence in written documents of subject expertise and critical awareness of the library's collections and its users, and demonstrate understanding of the library's collection policies? These factors grow in importance as the proportion of the position devoted to collection activities and the level of responsibility increases. For the librarian whose major responsibility is to manage or coordinate collection development, the assessment should also include such questions as what contributions has the person made to the profession—through professional activity, research, or writing.

Measuring Effectiveness

Ultimately the measure of a collection selector's or manager's effectiveness is how well the collection serves its purpose. Are the right materials available at the right time? Are information needs met well? Are users happy with the collection? Analysis of interlibrary loan requests, availability studies to assess whether the library owns or provides prompt access to the materials sought, citation studies to measure how many of the works that local researchers cite in their own publications are owned by the library, and satisfaction surveys are methods that can be used to judge how well the collections serve the library's clientele. Each method has its drawbacks and may measure factors other than success or failure in collection development. Nevertheless, collection assessment always reflects collection development performance, both past and present.

Sources for Performance Appraisal

A number of sources can be used to assess how well a librarian is carrying out collection responsibilities. These include self-evaluations, project reports, budget documents, reviews from peers, lists of accomplishments and progress reports on goals, comments from users or colleagues outside the library. Some helpful suggestions, and even formats for review, can be found in the ARL SpecKit on "Performance Appraisal of Collection Development Librarians" [9].

Relationship to Education

Performance appraisal should be viewed both as a training tool and a professional development mechanism. For this reason it is covered in this chapter on education rather than in Chapter 2, Roles and Relationships in Collection Management. Assessment of work is a management responsibility; it is also the individual's responsibility. Its purpose is to assure that the individual develops collections responsive to user needs. Effective management of collection development should result in effective collections. Good training, continuing education, and periodic performance assessment are all means for achieving this goal.

References

1. Woodsworth A, Lester J. Educational imperatives of the future research library: a symposium. J Acad Libr 1991 Sep; 17(4):204-15.

2. Metz P. Collection development in the library and information science curriculum. In: Johnson P, Intner SS. Recruiting, educating, and training librarians for collection development. Westport, CT: Greenwood Press, 1994: 87-97.

3. Steig MF. Change and challenge in library and information science education. Chicago: American Library Association, 1992: 109.

4. Johnson P. Collection development is more than selecting a title: education for a variety of responsibilities. In: Johnson P, Intner SS. Recruiting, educating, and training librarians for collection development. Westport, CT: Greenwood Press, 1994: 113-26.

5. Creth SD. Effective on-the-job training: developing library human resources. Chicago, American Library Association, 1986.

6. Guide for writing a bibliographer's manual. Chicago: American Library Association, 1987. (Collection management and development guides, no. 1).

7. Collection development organization and staffing in ARL libraries. Washington, DC: Office of Management Studies, Association of Research Libraries, Feb. 1987. (SPEC Kit no. 131).

8. Contempo 1995. JAMA. 1996 Jun 19;275(23):1791-1858.

9. Performance appraisal of collection development librarians. Washington, DC: Office Management Studies. Association of Research Libraries, Feb 1992. (SPEC Kit no. 181).

4

Policies and Criteria

"Few would doubt that a library's policy statement on collection development and management is a Good Thing (capital G, capital T)."
G. Edward Evans, 1985

"Collection development policies as traditionally conceived are static, reactive, and of little practical utility. They have outlived their purpose."
Dan Hazen, 1995

As the library's mission, objectives, and goals should reflect those of its parent institution, so too should the library's collection development program reflect the institution. The information needs of components of the institution that are served by the library, for example, should figure prominently in the collection development effort. The scope of the collection development program should parallel the extent of the institutional commitment to various activities and disciplines. The collection development program should reflect the very character of its parent institution. Except in the case of very specialized libraries, it is not possible for a library to have in its local collection everything that its users might potentially need. To provide a context within which to make choices, there must be stated goals and objectives for collection development. These must be derived from a conscious assessment of the information needs of the library user group. Ideally, the goals of a collection development program should be an extension of a long-range plan for the library.

In general, financial support for collections in health sciences libraries has declined during the recent past although the number of in-scope titles being published continues to increase. Information is being packaged in new and multiple formats as well. Recent significant changes in the environment for library services have greatly expanded the concept of access and made it a key concern of the public services agenda and the collection development program in most health sciences libraries. These factors have caused libraries to develop more rigorous selection methodologies and also to define more closely the criteria and processes by which decisions are made. A decision to acquire a journal title, for example, carries with it a future commitment of funds for binding and staff time for processing; such mortgages on the future typically require that libraries adhere to a systematic set of policies and criteria for journal selection. Redundancy of information and publication in multiple formats place added requirements on the drafting of policies and the application of criteria so that decisions are made in an informed manner.

That collection development policies are important to libraries was not always the case, nor indeed were they always necessary. Prior to the "information explosion" when many libraries felt that it was still possible for them to acquire everything published, or at least everything within a defined area, there was little need to articulate policies to govern the process. For many of the same reasons that acquisitions evolved into collection development, there has been a gradual recognition of the value of documenting the policies and procedures that surround collection development.

Atkinson, in an especially perceptive essay on collection development policies, observed that communication is the primary purpose of those policies [1]. A policy statement facilitates communication between a library and its user groups and within the library itself. To be an effective communication tool, a policy statement should provide an accurate description of the current state of the collection and it should contain strategies to facilitate the selection process. Last, the policy statement is tangible evidence that a systematic collection plan exists [2].

The debate has shifted from the need for documentation to the type of documentation. Hazen proposes that collection development librarians should consider replacing extensive policy documents with "flexible descriptions that encompass all formats of information and resources both local and remote" [3]. These flexible descriptions will require continuous revision as each field's methods and materials evolve in today's rapidly changing health care environment.

Recommended guidelines for collection development policies in health sciences libraries are contained in a MLA DocKit published in 1992 [4]. The American Library Association issued a pamphlet which contains useful and pertinent information for writing collection development policies [5]. Futas' *Collection Development Policies and Procedures* [6] and Gabriel's *Collection Development and Assessment* [7] provide additional guidance and examples of policy statements. Finally, Dowd's classic paper on drafting collection development policies, though published more than a decade ago, still has merit [8].

Rationales for Documentation of Policy

There are many reasons to draft a collection development policy and those which apply will vary from institution to institution. Its use as a communication vehicle has already been discussed. The following list, based on Evans [9] and Eakin [10] contains additional reasons to document the policy and the process.

- To relate the goals of the library to the goals of the institution.
- To provide a rational basis for selection, deselection, and preservation decision making.
- To demonstrate that collections are developed to support specific institutional programs.
- To assure that the needs of the inarticulate and reticent will be served, as well as those of the articulate and vocal.
- To establish a framework for budget allocations and to lend legitimacy to those allocations.
- To communicate to users and other institutions the nature and limits of the collection.
- To be a vehicle for focusing attention on the library—either from outside sources such as donors, or inside sources such as administrators.
- To assign responsibility for collection development and define relationships among staff and with other libraries or institutions.
- To promote consistency in collection development decision making and to minimize "individual" interpretation of policies.
- To educate staff and users to the importance of collection development and its place within the library.
- To ensure that the collection stays current.
- To serve as a benchmark for collection assessment and evaluation studies.
- To provide a base for long-range planning.
- To articulate criteria which govern collection development.

A critical step for the librarian to take early in the drafting of a collection development policy is to articulate the reasons for preparing such a document in the particular library. These reasons should be discussed with colleagues. In this way the documentation process can be more easily adjusted to fit the specific needs of the library.

Elements of Collection Development Policies

Policy statements range from a single page to large manuals, generally reflecting the size of the institution and its constituencies or the degree of interest of the library staff in drafting such policies. There is no magic formula for collection development policy writing, nor is there a prescribed form that all policies must follow. This fact is readily apparent in the excerpts from actual policy statements and a small representative collection of complete hospital library collection development policy statements which appear in Appendix A.

It is recommended that librarians contemplating the writing of a collection development policy turn to examples for inspiration and for emulation. This can greatly speed the documentation process. Many libraries, including NLM, will make their policy statements available in electronic form, facilitating the writing process even more.

This section describes the basic elements which should be considered for inclusion in a collection development policy.

Introduction

An introductory section sets the tone for the policy to follow. It should include the institutional and library mission; a list of institutional programs supported by the library; a description of the user group; a brief history of the collection; notes on cooperative agreements, formal and informal; relationships with other libraries; and an indication of sources used by the library to stay abreast of the programs of the institution. Some form of review and approval cycle for the policy should be included to ensure that the document stays current and useful.

Definitions and Responsibilities

This section contains definitions of terms used, responsibilities for collection development, and general principles which guide collection development processes. It is important to define collecting levels in order to establish a common understanding and use of terms such as "research," "comprehensive," and others. National organizations such as ALA and the Research Libraries Group (RLG) have attempted from time to time to standardize these definitions across all types of libraries, with some success. In 1988, the RLG issued a set of definitions for collecting levels to be used by health sciences libraries participating in the RLG Conspectus, a national online inventory of collections of RLG participating institutions [11]. These definitions appear in Table 4-1.

Many health sciences libraries use the RLG or other definitions to describe collecting levels. NLM modified the RLG definitions in earlier editions of its collection development policy. In the 1993 edition of its *Collection Development Manual*, NLM ceased the practice of using several collecting levels to define its collection development program and devised the following description of collecting.

In order to fulfill its mandate to its defined user community, NLM attempts to assemble a comprehensive collection of the research and professional biomedical literature, broadly defined. NLM's concept of comprehensive collecting is compatible with the Comprehensive level defined by the Research Libraries Group (RLG).

Comprehensive Level: A collection in which a library endeavors, so far as reasonably possible, to include all significant works of recorded knowledge (publications, manuscripts, other forms) in all applicable languages, for a necessarily defined and limited field. This level of collecting intensity is one that maintains a "special collection"; the aim, if not the achievement, is exhaustiveness. Older material is retained for historical research. The scope of the NLM collection, encompassing as it does all of biomedicine, is significantly broader than is generally understood for the "special collection" referred to in the RLG definition. NLM recognizes that while it is possible to assemble a collection which addresses all topics in biomedicine, it is impossible even for a national library to gather a complete, worldwide collection of all biomedical materials in all formats. The section, "Special Considerations in Selection," presents strategies for identifying and selecting particular types of materials in order to allow NLM to approach, insofar as possible, the ideal of a comprehensive collection in biomedicine [12].

Selection Criteria

This section defines the factors taken into account and assessed in the selection process. Additional detail follows in a separate part of this chapter.

Table 4-1: Research Libraries Group Definitions for Collecting Levels

Out of Scope

The library does not collect in this area.

Minimal Level

A subject area in which few selections are made beyond very basic works.

Basic Information Level

A highly selective collection which serves to introduce and define the subject, and to indicate the varieties of information available elsewhere. It includes a representative selection of dictionaries, encyclopedias, historical surveys, access to appropriate bibliographic data bases, bibliographies, and handbooks, in the minimum number that will serve the purpose. It contains selected editions of textbooks and monographs and the periodicals cited in the Brandon-Hill list. A basic information collection is not sufficiently intensive to support any advanced undergraduate or graduate courses or independent study in the subject area involved.

Instructional Support Level

A selective collection which is adequate to support undergraduate and MOST graduate instruction, or sustained independent study within a curriculum, and health care in a hospital or clinical setting; that is, a collection which is adequate to maintain knowledge of a subject required for limited or generalized purposes, of less than research intensity. It includes the major reference tools for the pertinent subject, significant indexing and abstracting services, access to appropriate non-bibliographic data bases, a broad selection of major textbooks, monographs, and government documents, and a wide range of basic periodicals, including at least 25% of the English language titles pertinent to the subject in *List of Journals Indexed in Index Medicus*.

Research Level

A collection which contains the major published source materials required for dissertations and independent research, including specialized reference tools, conference proceedings, professional society publications, technical reports, government documents, multiple editions of most textbooks and monographs, including a significant number of titles pertinent to the subject in a recognized "standard" bibliography, an extensive collection of periodicals, including at least 65% of the titles pertinent to the subject in *List of Journals Indexed in Index Medicus*. While English materials may predominate, the collection usually contains important materials in French, German, Spanish, Russian, and other languages. Older or superseded materials are retained for historical research.

Comprehensive Level

A collection in which the library endeavors, insofar as possible, to include all significant works of recorded knowledge (publications, manuscripts, other forms) in all applicable languages for a necessarily defined and limited field. This level of collecting intensity is one that maintains a "special collection" the aim, if not the achievement, is exhaustiveness.

Subjects

A subject outline with definitions and an indication of exclusions and special emphases sets the scope for the collecting effort.

Formats

A section dealing with formats and any particular policies or principles that affect their selection provides guidance for publication types such as pamphlets, theses, and others.

Special Policies

This section contains policy and sometimes procedural statements on such issues as donated items, multiple copies, replacements, retention, preservation, and collection evaluation.

Special Settings

Archival and historical collection policies, policies for reference collections, audiovisual collections, consumer health collections are compiled in this section. Additional detail on these appears in Chapter 7, Selection in Special Settings.

Writing the Policy

A collection development policy should contain the pertinent documentation or references to that documentation that influence and guide collection development processes, especially selection and deselection. The preceding outline provides a basic framework within which to organize appropriate documentation.

Responsibility for the writing of collection development policy will vary from institution to institution. Policy formulation and review can originate from within the library, from a governing board, from within the user group, or from other outside groups with a vested interest. It is in the library's interest to initiate the process and to see it through to completion. A review of existing statements and some background work, coupled with a review of statements from libraries in similar institutions will provide the necessary background data from which to develop a draft. The draft should be circulated among library staff, and comment from library users should be sought. Ultimately the document is referred to a governing authority. Once a draft has been approved, the document should be shared widely. Among the most important segments of the policy statement is a description of the criteria that guide collection development.

Selection Criteria

Selection criteria are the factors taken into account by the librarian in determining whether or not to add a particular item to a collection. The following criteria and guidelines form the basis for the selection process in any health sciences library. These criteria apply to all materials but may assume greater or lesser importance depending on the type of material under consideration. Also, other criteria may be important in special instances. The conscientious application of an accepted set of criteria allows the library to reaffirm in current terms its goal to provide a collection appropriate for present and future users; it also allows for the judicious expenditure of available funds. The selection process should be a weighing of these factors, one against or with another, to reach a decision.

Need and Potential Use

The concept of need or potential use has been a basic tenet of the collection development process and consequently a fundamental selection criterion for much of library history. It is the *sine qua non* of selection. Predictions of use are best made based on a solid knowledge of the user group. A collection development policy should include an up-to-date listing of the schools, departments, and institutes that comprise the library's primary and secondary user groups; this list should be consulted with regularity in the selection process. The list should be augmented with a general description of the needs of constituencies, and any other important information such as research activities, grants, and special clinical programs. Maintenance of such a list allows the library both to anticipate and to provide for changing needs within the user group. In recent years, there has been a pronounced shift from predictive or anticipatory buying to on-demand purchasing in response to a demonstrated need.

Scope and Content of the Item

What is the purpose of the item? Is it likely to be of interest to only a few individuals or is it something of interest to all library users? Does the item address a basic topic, such as anatomy, or a surgical or diagnostic procedure? Or is the topic of no particular lasting interest? Preference is generally given to items that are of sufficient breadth to be of use and interest to a department or to an interdisciplinary program that cuts across departmental lines. Materials of interest to programs limited to a small number of individuals or requests from individuals should certainly be considered and selected, but in relation to more comprehensive titles.

Quality

There are two quality types—content and technical—both of which are subjective.

Content

Content quality is best determined by weighing several factors collectively; those factors include sponsorship, comprehensiveness, relevance, the degree of scholarship, the immediate value of the information in context or the lasting value of the item itself, the reputations of the author, publisher, the contributors, the editorial board, the producers, the authority of the information presented; and the impact of the title in the discipline, especially important for journals. Also of increasing importance in the selection of journals is evidence of peer review.

Technical

Technical quality reflects the type and amount of illustration, bibliographies, clarity of images, the type of binding and paper. In the case of audiovisuals, one considers the cinematography and production details, sound quality, quality of video or audiotape. Acid-free paper and preservability of the physical pieces are of growing importance in the selection process. None of these should be the deciding factor alone but each should be considered as it contributes to or detracts from the overall quality of the item.

Depth of the Existing Collection

It will rarely be necessary for a library to acquire all the titles that may be of interest; existing strengths of the collection should be considered as should overlaps in collecting responsibility and collections with other nearby libraries. Further, other items on the topic already in the collection should be assessed to determine if they can meet the need. Availability of the title through extramural formal and informal arrangements, while less important than availability within the local institution, should be considered. Affiliations should be noted as well as cooperative acquisition programs in which the library participates. Cooperation generally allows the library to minimize purchase of titles for which low demand may exist. The net result is an increase in the available information base within the consortium.

Currency, Timeliness, Uniqueness

Clinical practice and continuing medical education in the health sciences require the most up-to-date information. Such information changes very rapidly. Preference is usually given to items which report new or revised information in a timely fashion or present a different perspective from something already in the collection. What is the publication date? Is the item of historical interest only?

Bibliographic Accessibility

Although this criterion applies principally to journal literature, it is included here because that literature is considered primary in health sciences libraries. The decision to include a journal in an indexing source increases access to its contents and also the level of use of the title in the library. Because libraries include in reference collections a large number of primary indexes and offer search access to online databases, bibliographic accessibility should be a primary criterion in the selection and retention of journal titles. Preference in many libraries may be given to titles included in such standard databases as MEDLINE and CINAHL. Journals in other sources, such as EMBASE and PsycINFO, may be given a lower selection priority. In other settings, these values may change.

Inclusion of Title in a Recommended List

The sponsorship of the item has already been noted under quality, but if the item is also on a recommended list (such as Brandon/Hill) or in a list from a health-related association for accreditation or for a particular continuing education activity, or if it appears on a list which has been systematically compiled, an item may have greater appeal, especially when there are several similar items from which to choose.

Audience Level of the Item

Is the item developed and published for the professional audience? For the intelligent lay audience? Is it for use in patient education or continuing medical education? What is the level of difficulty of the item? Can several types of library users or health professionals benefit from using the item?

Price

Price, whether high or low, should rarely be the sole criterion in deciding whether or not to select a given item. It should be considered in relation to more primary criteria or in comparison to costs of other similar works.

Language and Country of Origin

Most libraries will indicate in a collection development policy if materials in languages other than English and titles published outside the United States are collected.

Specialized Formats and Environments

The above criteria form the basis for the selection process in any library. They are generic in that they have applicability across formats and subjects. The criteria that are considered in selection decision making have become more and more detailed over time, and, when selection decisions are being made for special formats (such as audiovisuals and computer software or for materials in special settings like rare book collections), additional factors are taken into account.

These general selection criteria apply also in hospital settings, but the following additional criteria may also figure prominently in a selection decision as well: 1) space to house item; 2) the clinical orientation of the information presented; 3) the availability of the item through affiliated institutions; 4) the appearance on a Brandon/Hill list; and 5) the types and presence of hospital services or clinical units, such as obstetrics ward, grief counseling service, drug rehabilitation unit, emergency room. Additional guidance can be gleaned from Hardy's discussion of the topic [13].

Application of Criteria

The selection process is defined as the application of selection criteria to an actual item under consideration for inclusion in a library collection. Chapters 5, 6, and 7 deal with this concept in a more comprehensive way for specific classes of materials, but the following coda has application in virtually all selection processes.

Ten Selection Principles

1. Use/demand/need, potential or immediate, is the most important criterion in making a selection decision.
2. Use/demand/need, potential or immediate, need not always be satisfied by inclusion of an item in the local collection.
3. The selection process is a weighing of the criterion of use/demand/need against all other criteria.
4. Assessment of quality is generally a subjective process, made less so through the consideration of other opinions such as expert opinion about periodicals selected for inclusion in indexes and reviewer opinions in peer-reviewed journals.
5. Newness or uniqueness are not inherently positive criteria for selection.
6. The price of a given item and its value in the library collection are not necessarily related.
7. Price should rarely be the sole criterion in a selection decision.
8. Access is as important as ownership for a growing class and number of library materials.
9. Selection is a private cognitive activity [14] for which experience is the best teacher.
10. Generous funding does not guarantee a high-quality collection [15].

This brief discussion of selection criteria demonstrates the range of criteria that health sciences libraries take into account in the selection process. These criteria are continually undergoing refinement in the local setting through application and as the selection process is adjusted to accommodate changing needs of library users. The complexity of scholarship, the increasing number of formats in which information is packaged, the continued splitting of fields, will each affect the selection process and the application of criteria. These factors and others will require ongoing analysis of potential additions to the collection at a greater level of specificity. Evans has said that "collection development was, is, and always will be subjective, biased work" [16]. By continually reviewing the criteria that comprise the selection process, librarians can reduce the degree of bias in that process [17].

References

1. Atkinson R. The language of the levels: reflections on the communication of collection development policy. Coll Res Libr 1986 Mar; 47(2):140-9.
2. American Library Association. Reference and Adult Services Division. Collection Development Policies Committee. The relevance of collection development policies: definition, necessity, and applications. RQ 1993 Fall;33(1):65-74.
3. Hazen D. Collection development policies in the information age. Coll Res Libr 1995 Jan;56(1):29-31.
4. Morse DH, Richards DT. Collection development policies for health sciences libraries. Chicago: Medical Library Association, 1992. (MLA DocKit no. 3).
5. Bryant B, ed. Guide for written collection policy statements. Chicago: American Library Association, 1989. (Collection management and development guides, no. 3).
6. Futas, E, ed. Collection development policies and procedures. 3rd ed. Phoenix, AZ: Oryx Press, 1995.
7. Gabriel D. Collection development and assessment. London: Scarecrow Press, 1995.
8. Dowd ST. The formulation of a collection development policy statement. In: Stueart RD, Miller GB, eds. Collection development in libraries: a treatise. v. 1. Greenwich, CT: JAI Press, 1980.
9. Evans GE. Developing library and information center collections. 2d ed. Littleton, CO: Libraries Unlimited, 1987.
10. Eakin D. Health science library materials: collection development. In Darling L, Bishop D, Colaianni LA, eds. Handbook of medical library practice. 4th ed. v. 2. Chicago, Medical Library Association 1983:27-91.
11. Richards DT. RLG conspectus supplemental guidelines for medical and health sciences. Stanford, CA: The Research Libraries Group, 1988:2.
12. Collection development manual of the National Library of Medicine. 3rd ed. Bethesda, MD: National Library of Medicine, 1993:3-4.
13. Hardy MC. Selection of library materials. In: Bradley J, Holst R, Messerle J, eds. Hospital library management. Chicago: Medical Library Association, 1983:29-44.
14. Atkinson, op. cit., 142.
15. Eakin, op. cit., 28.
16. Evans, op. cit., 20.
17. Richards DT. By your selection criteria are ye known. Libr Acq Pract Theory 1991;15 (3):279-85.

5

Selection: Journals and Books

"What are countless books to me, and libraries which the owner in his whole life will scarcely read the titles?"

Seneca

Selection requires judgment about what materials are relevant to the institution's purpose, useful to the library's clientele, and meet standards for content quality. Journals and books will be considered in this chapter. Electronic journals are discussed here; other electronic resources are addressed in Chapter 6, Selection: Electronic Resources. Special purpose collections—reference, audiovisual and multi-media, patient education, rare books, and archives—are covered in Chapter 7, Selection in Special Settings.

Journal Selection

From the eighteenth century, the journal has been an important mechanism for communicating scientific findings, advances in techniques, and changes in accepted practice in medicine and other health professions. As we approach the twenty-first century, journals remain one of the most essential methods for conveying new knowledge in the health sciences, though there are indications that this role will change in the near future. Peer-reviewed journals also constitute the accepted method for establishing primacy of discovery and documenting scholarly contributions for promotion, tenure, and professional advancement. Journals continue to constitute the core of health sciences library collections and, except for personnel costs, journal subscriptions account for the largest segment of the library's budget.

Many new biomedical journals appear each year, despite the inability of libraries to keep up with price increases, the dwindling number of personal and institutional subscribers to high-priced journals, and the threat that print publications will be overshadowed by electronic forms of scientific communication. Both interdisciplinary and ultraspecialized publications emerge or split off from existing journals. This trend is likely to continue as long as scientists are rewarded for publishing their research and institutions gain recognition and prestige through the disseminated writings of their faculty.

The Process

Responsibility

Each library must determine who is responsible for journal selection, how many individuals or groups will play a part in the process, and with whom the final decision rests. Several possible models for distributing collection responsibilities are outlined in Chapter 2, Roles and Relationships in Collection Development. Because a decision to subscribe to a journal is often a long-term one, with a financial commitment over several years, selection is rarely left to a single person, although the final determination to acquire a title often lies in the hands of the library director or collection manager.

Selection Committees

In academic health sciences libraries and in large hospital libraries, a committee approach works well. Suggestions or requests for new subscriptions are brought to the group for review. Criteria for evaluating titles are agreed upon and an evaluation form is used to collect data for decision making and to document decisions. Periodically the group meets to review titles under consideration. In the days of generous budgets, such reviews might have been conducted monthly, and in settings where an institutional advisory committee is directly involved in selection, decisions may still be made on a monthly or bimonthly basis. However, less frequent reviewing offers a number of advantages:

- More titles will be evaluated at the same time, allowing reviewers to rank titles in priority order, using limited funds for the highest priority titles.

- There is a greater chance that there will be multiple new journals in the same or overlapping disciplines, stimulating critical comparisons.
- Quarterly or semiannual reviews of potential new subscriptions may also permit more extensive data gathering to compare new journals with existing subscriptions in the same field or to solicit input from a wider range of potential users.
- With more elapsed time between reviews, additional data on interlibrary loan requests or user need may be also accumulated.
- If new orders are placed only once or twice a year, it may be preferable for decisions on new subscriptions to coincide with the order and renewal process.

Regardless of the frequency with which decisions are made, the individual or group making final recommendations should be provided with adequate information on which to base a judgment. Useful information for reviewers would include

- Title.
- Publisher.
- Frequency.
- Starting date.
- Cost.
- Coverage of contents by standard indexing and abstracting services and online databases.
- Published rankings or reviews.
- Interlibrary loan data.
- Information about purchase requests.
- Information about other titles in the subject field.
- Evidence of peer review of articles.
- Assessments by faculty or hospital staff.
- Availability in other affiliated libraries.
- Relevance to institutional programs.

This information should be recorded in a consistent manner on a standard form to allow those making decisions to make comparisons more easily. Figures 5-1 and 5-2 include some representative forms.

Journal/Book Recommendation
Cushing/Whitney Medical Library
Yale University

Your Name .... Date ....
Department .... Status ....
Campus Address ....
University/Hospital Identification Number _ _ _-_ _-_ _ _ _ Telephone Number (_ _ _) _ _ _-_ _ _ _

Please attach a copy of advertisement or other related information if available.

Journal

Journal subscriptions are reviewed on a regular basis for both additions and cancellations.   You will be notified of the final decision.

Title ....
Publisher .... Price ....
Comments *(e.g. Are there other important titles in the same discipline? What is the importance or impact of this journal?*
Are there other journals currently received which could be cancelled if we subscribed to this journal?): ....
....
....
....
....
....

Book

Author/Editor ....
Title ....
Publisher .... Edition/Volume ....
Place of publication .... Price ....

Would you like to have the book held for your use upon its receipt?   Yes ....   No ....

Figure 5-1: Journal/Book Recommendation (Yale University)

Staff Use Only

Journals	Books
ORBIS ___ Medical ___ Other	ORBIS ___ Medical ___ Other ....
___ LTLC ___ SERLINE	___ LTLC ___ RLIN
ISSN	ISBN ....
Indexing/Abstracting ___ MEDLINE ___ PsycInfo ___ SCI ___ BIOSIS ___ CCON ___ CINAHL ___ INI ___ HEALTHLINE ___ Excerpta Medica ___ Other	Notes: ....
Patron Notified/Request .... ILL Requests .... SCI Impact Factor .... RLIN/OCLC .... Reinstatement/Date Cancelled? .... First Year of Title	
Yale Editor(s) .... Yale Author(s)	
Notes	
Request Sample Issue .... Date Sample Ordered .... Decision .... Initiate Subscription With .... Fund Code .... Patron Notified/Final	Fund Code .... Patron Notified ....

Left margin labels:

Book — Orbis # .... Date .... Decision ....

Journal — Title .... Date .... Decision ....

recommendation form/collection development/pm5 8-94

Figure 5-1: Journal/ Book Recommendation, Verso (Yale University)

SUGGESTED JOURNAL FOR UTHSCSA COLLECTION

JOURNAL CONSIDERED FOR   ( ) ADD   ( ) CANCEL   DATE _____

TITLE: _____

PUBLISHER: _____

PRICE: _____   FREQUENCY: _____   BEGAN PUBLICATION: _____

RECOMMENDED BY: _____ DEPT: _____
( ) Acknowledged   ( ) Unsolicited mail   ( ) Publisher's announcement
( ) ILL copyright limit reached: ___Covered   ___ Not covered by CCC

FACULTY EVALUATION
Reviewer: _____   Rating: _____ Reviewer: _____Rating: _____

Reviewer: _____   Rating: _____Reviewer: _____Rating: ____

San Antonio library holdings: _____

SCAMeL library holdings: _____

ILL history: _____

Indexed by: _____

Comparison with related journals in the collection:

Title	Price	Impact Factor (#citations/# articles)						Index
This title								
1.								
2.								
3.								
4.								
5.								
6.								
7.								

SERIALS REVIEW COMMITTEE COMMENTS (Use reverse for extensive comments)
Suggested options: ❏ Add   ❏ Do not add
                        ❏ Purchase backfiles   ❏ Cancel subscription
                        ❏ Withdraw holdings   ❏ Sample file
Director: _____

Asst. Dir Public Services: _____

Reference Librarian: _____

Monographs Selection Officer: _____

Asst Dir Collection Dev: _____

ILL Librarian: _____
( ) REQUESTOR NOTIFIED OF DECISION
BEGIN WITH: _____
LOCATION: ( ) Briscoe   ( ) Brady/Green   ( ) _____
ACCOUNT: _____ , __ VENDOR: _____ VENDOR TITLE #_____
SUBJECT HEADINGS _____
BACKFILE PURCHASE: ( ) No   ( ) Yes   Begin with _____
REPORTED TO:
SCAMeL ULS: _____ COLLECTION DEV: _____
CORAL ULS: _____ COLLECTION DEV: _____

Figure 5-2: Journal Recommendation Form (University of Texas Health Science Center at San Antonio)

External Reviewers

If faculty or other health professional staff are involved in the evaluation of new journals, but do not participate in group decision making, the library may want to gather their opinions as new titles are proposed throughout the year. Individuals given only an occasional journal to evaluate may be more willing to offer critical comment than if confronted with several titles at one time.

To get maximum benefit from their expertise, the library must protect its consultants' time. A journal evaluation form to be used by faculty or clinical staff can be tailored to elicit opinion on specific characteristics of each journal. Basic information should be provided, including many of the items listed previously. If at all possible, a sample issue should be obtained prior to faculty review and shared with the reviewer. While it may be easier for reviewers to simply check off a box rating the journal in terms of content, quality, and importance to current departmental needs, they should also be encouraged to write critical comments. Electronic communication may also be used to transmit evaluations. Sample issues need to be clearly marked so they are returned, especially if the library wants opinions from more than one source. However, expectations should be tempered by the realization that no matter what tactics are used, some issues will not come back and some responses will be perfunctory.

If the library uses departmental representatives to assist in journal selection, the expectations for the representatives should be clearly communicated. When these consultants are asked to review a new journal, they need to understand whether they are being asked for their own opinion and their interpretation of departmental needs, or whether they are expected to actively survey their department. It may be best to convey the importance of representing department needs, but leave the mechanism for soliciting additional opinions up to the representative. Large departments will often encompass multiple areas of specialization and the representative may simply refer the evaluation to an expert in the specialty, rather than routing the journal to the entire department. Alternatively, the library may invite the representative to suggest additional reviewers known to work in the particular specialty. The library may then follow up to get further opinions.

Record Keeping

In larger libraries that review and make decisions on many titles, a record-keeping system that tracks reviews in progress and completed decisions is helpful. A card file or a manual file of review forms are the simplest approaches. However, when many titles are reviewed, an automated file using database management software may more easily keep track of information and allow searching by specific element, such as title, publisher, or follow-up date. Data to be kept in such a database might include

- Title.
- Publisher.
- Subject area.
- Frequency.
- Cost.
- Date sample was requested/received; follow up dates.
- Selector name.
- External reviewer name.
- Date review was requested/received; follow up dates.
- Rating.
- Purchase decision.
- Institutional program or unit supported.
- Fund.

With a database, information about the number of journals reviewed over a period of time, the number rejected, reason for rejection, costs, and other factors can be extracted and analyzed. Such data are useful in budget preparation, reporting to the institutional administration, and even newsletter articles to inform the library's clientele about publishing trends and library collection decisions. The library's automated system may also be able to track some or all of the desired data.

Sources of Information

Information about new journals may be found in various sources.

Advertising and Announcements

Ads are frequently sent directly by the publisher or are published in library or medical journals. Vendors alert libraries to new titles in various ways, through lists, order forms, and online information systems. Catalogs from publishers may also be used to identify new journals.

Sample Issues

Publishers may send unsolicited samples or trial issues. More often a sample issue must be requested and sometimes purchased.

Core Lists

Lists of key journals have been compiled for specialized fields and may be useful, especially if the library is to take on support for a new program. Examples are listed in Table 5-1.

User Recommendations

The library can encourage user suggestions by making request forms prominently available in the library, soliciting recommendations through a library newsletter, electronic bulletin board, Web home page, or by asking departments directly. Electronic mail may be an easy way for users to send requests to the library, especially if a request format is a menu choice on the institution's communications network. Request forms should specify the critical data elements needed such as title, publisher, or publication date.

Interlibrary Loan Requests

Repeated requests from users to obtain articles from a journal should prompt the library to consider a subscription. An alerting process, whether it is initiated from automated records or paper files should be used to identify journals which are being requested frequently from other libraries. Libraries with significant borrowing activity will need a more formal and systematic process than libraries with light borrowing activity. The library should establish a threshold, such as the guideline of five suggested by the CONTU Guidelines, which, when reached, triggers an alert to the person responsible for collection development. That title should then be considered in the established review process.

Reviews

Reviews of scientific journals are harder to come by than book reviews, but some sources do exist. *Nature* annually publishes an issue in which new journals in the basic sciences are critically reviewed and since 1992 *JAMA* has published evaluative reviews of new journals in clinical medicine [1-2]. Targeted more specifically for librarians, *Serials Review* regularly includes reviews of journals [3]. Although excluding clinical medicine, these reviews do encompass the physical, social, and life sciences. As decisions on journal subscriptions are often not made immediately, journal reviews may be more useful to libraries than book reviews.

Table 5-1: Selected Core Lists

Medical

Brandon AN, Hill DR. Selected list of books and journals for the small medical library. Bull Med Libr Assoc 1995 Apr;83(2):151-75.
Hague H, comp. Core collection of medical books and journals. 2d ed. London: Medical Information Working Party, 1994.
Mazza JJ. A library for internists VIII. Recommendations from the American College of Physicians. Ann Intern Med 1994 Apr 15;120(8):699-720.
Recommended book list for family practice residency libraries. Kansas City, MO: American Academy of Family Physicians, 1995.
Slater BM, Slater MA. Determining core journals in behavioral medicine. Bull Med Libr Assoc 1994 Jul;84(3):289-309,

Nursing and Allied Health

Brandon AN, Hill DR. Selected list of books and journals in allied health. Bull Med Libr Assoc 1996 Jul; 84(3):289-309.
Brandon AN, Hill DR. Selected list of nursing books and journals. Nurs Outlook 1996 Mar/Apr; 44(2):56-66.
Interagency Council on Library Resources for Nursing. Essential nursing references. Amer J Nurs 1992 Sep; 92(9):83-4, 86, 88, 90.
Murphy SC. Nursing research journals: a discussion and annotated guide. Ser Rev 1993 Summer; 19(2):23-8.

Dentistry

Johnson RC, Mason F, Sims RH. A basic list of recommended books and journals for support of clinical dentistry in a non-dental library. Developed by the Ad Hoc Committee of the Dental Section of the Medical Library Association, 1996.

Veterinary

Boyd CT et al. Basic list of veterinary serials. 2nd ed. 1981, with revisions to April 1, 1986. Ser Libr 1986 Oct; 11(2)5-39.

Indexes

Lists of journals indexed for major indexing services, such as MEDLINE, *Current Contents*, BIOSIS, and CINAHL are used more often to make a judgment on journals already identified. However, announcements of journals added to any of these databases can be used to alert selectors to titles that have met certain criteria and, because they will be retrieved on searches, may be in greater demand. Journals added to MEDLINE are announced in *The NLM Technical Bulletin* and newly added titles to *Current Contents* are listed at the front of its issues [4-5].

Applying Collection Policy

The library's collection policy and selection criteria should guide the selection of journals as well as books. The subject scope and depth of local collections, as described in Chapter 4, Policies and Criteria, apply to all media types—for electronic as well as print publications. Criteria for journal selection, however, must take into account the unique characteristics of the journal format.

Quality

The quality of a publication is a prime consideration in deciding whether to subscribe, but how does the librarian judge quality in a journal? No single measure will be sufficient; reviewers must take into account numerous factors and ask a range of questions.

Publisher

Who is responsible for the publication? If the journal is issued by a commercial publisher, consider its reputation as a scientific publisher. Look at other journals from the same publisher to determine the quality of printing, illustrations, paper, and binding. Does the publisher maintain a regular publication schedule, avoiding extra volumes or unannounced supplements? While these factors may not be indicative of the quality of the articles, they may have considerable impact on costs and timeliness. If the publisher is known for producing journals with refereed and highly cited articles, its new journals are likely to follow the same pattern.

Is the journal published by or for a professional society or association? If so, does the organization represent a major discipline or esoteric subspecialty? Is its membership international, primarily national, or does it reflect the interests of a regional group? A new journal sponsored by a professional society often reflects a perceived need for scientific communication within the discipline, a desire to draw together articles focusing on a particular clinical subspecialty, a new diagnostic or therapeutic technique, or interdisciplinary research that has grown in importance.

Editors

Editors exercise control over the quality of articles published. If the editors are not recognized and institutional affiliations are not listed, one way to find out more about them is to determine whether they are themselves authors. Do they have articles indexed in MEDLINE? An editor who has contributed knowledge to the field should be qualified to make good judgments about scope and quality of articles submitted to the journal. A journal's editorial board may, and often does, include prominent names in the field, but it is not always clear what role they play with respect to the articles accepted for publication. Presumably such individuals would not lend their names to a publication if they doubted its quality, but a decision to subscribe should not be weighted heavily by names on the editorial board, unless of course they happen to include leading individuals in the local institution.

Editorial Review

The editorial review process may be an indicator of content quality. Articles subjected to peer review are expected to meet certain standards for research methods, data analysis, and accuracy. A study of English-language journals indexed in *Index Medicus* found that only half indicated a peer review practice [6]. When a journal does not state its practice, a request for the author to submit multiple copies often indicates the article will be distributed for external review. If the journal does not indicate peer review and there is no other evidence to suggest that such review is conducted, it may be useful to inquire. While reviews and didactic articles are more likely to be invited by the editor, and even paid for, they may still undergo a review process.

Authors

By examining sample issues, the selector will get a feeling for the quality of authorship in a journal. If papers are repeatedly authored by members of the editorial board, one might wonder whether the journal is having difficulty attracting submissions. If the journal's intent is to be international, the authors should represent a broad range of countries. Evaluating articles on the basis of the author's affiliation is risky. Scientific journals have been criticized for bias in selecting papers from prestigious institutions, but such bias has not been demonstrated [7]. However, if few articles in a journal that publishes original research emanate from major institutions with a reputation for clinical or basic research, the general content quality may be questioned. Further questions may be raised when authors' institutional affiliations are not given at all. One can ascertain publication experience by conducting an author search in MEDLINE or other sources.

Content—Research Journals

Research journals should publish articles that follow the accepted format for describing scientific research, giving the reader adequate background on the purpose of the study, full description of methods, clear presentation of results, analysis and discussion of significance. Research design should include adequate study populations, proper controls, and appropriate statistical analysis.

Content—Clinical Journals

Clinical practice journals may be more difficult for the librarian to judge and selection may depend more heavily on evaluation by practitioners. A series of articles prepared by the Evidence-Based Medicine Working Group provides a primer on evaluating articles, useful for librarians as well as practitioners [8-15]. The primary purpose of the clinical literature is to improve patient care, through better prevention, diagnosis, and treatment of disease. Articles reporting applied clinical research should describe the intervention, analyze the consequences, or discuss the implications, including benefits or disadvantages. A new clinical journal should be compared with existing publications covering the same topics to be certain that it offers more, different, or better information. Case reports, except for unique or unusual cases, should analyze a large series or cover a significant time period. When clinical journals attempt to serve multiple types of communication (scientist to scientist, scientist to practitioner, practitioner to practitioner, and practitioner to scientist) they may fail to serve the clinician well. Haynes has suggested a number of ways to improve standards in clinical journals [16].

Content—Review Journals

Reviews serve a special purpose. For house officers in particular, reviews can save precious time by bringing together much of the current information on a topic, eliminating the effort required to identify and digest the primary literature scattered among many journals. For practitioners, reviews may serve as a means of keeping up in fields that are outside their own specialty. And for researchers, reviews can provide a valuable introduction to a field that has taken on relevance for their work. Review articles may be published occasionally or regularly in journals that also publish original research; in addition, journals that are wholly devoted to reviews abound, representing almost every discipline and specialty.

Review journals require even more selectivity than research or practice journals because as secondary sources they are not reporting new information and reviews on similar topics may cover much of the same ground. While multiple journals in neurology may be needed, multiple review journals in neurology would be hard to justify. Reviews that cover a substantial topic, not merely enumerating past publications but synthesizing and critically appraising the field should be sought. Good reviews present the best of what is known at the time and discuss the controversies associated with the current state of knowledge or practice. Reviews by experts who can summarize and interpret in an expressive and readable style are cherished.

How does one judge a review journal? Several questions may guide the selector in making decisions. Is the subject scope broad enough for the contents to appeal to a range of users or is the scope focused on a narrow subspecialty that would be encompassed by other, more broadly aimed review journals? Are the writers authorities in their fields? Do the reviews cover topics comprehensively, highlight the most significant information, present multiple viewpoints when there is disagreement among experts, offer critical commentary? Are the reviews up-to-date? Allowing for publication lag time, do they cover important recent findings and are the references current and accurate? Is the writing eloquent or at least graceful?

Writing and Style

Although writing quality is a less critical element than authoritativeness and content, organization, readability, and adherence to standards for abstracts and references are good indicators of a journal's quality.

Writing Style

Articles should be readable. The writing should be grammatically correct, well organized, and clear. Poorly organized and poorly written articles are evidence of negligent or incompetent editing and also call into question the ability of the author.

Abstracts

Most substantive research and clinical journals now demand informative abstracts, which describe the major content of the article. A prescribed format for structured abstracts pioneered in *Annals of Internal Medicine* is common in many journals [17]. Structured abstracts concisely summarize the main points of the objective, design, setting, research subjects, intervention, main outcome measure, results, and conclusion.

References

Bibliographies should be pertinent, thorough, and up-to-date. Citations should be complete and accurate.

Accessibility of Content

One factor to consider in making a decision about a journal is how potential readers will be alerted to articles published in it. Although personal subscriptions, citations in articles, and references received from colleagues, are heavily relied upon by scientists, retrieval from searches of discipline-specific databases, such as MEDLINE, or tables-of-contents services are also significant [18]. Therefore, for journals that have been published for at least two or three years, accessibility through indexes may be a criterion for selection. Common sources for indexing information are *Ulrichs International Periodicals Directory*, SERLINE, and *The Serials Directory* [19-21], although all three sources tend to underreport coverage [22]. The National Library of Medicine's *List of Serials Indexed for Online Users* identifies journals covered by NLM's databases [23].

The inclusion of a journal in a selective database may also be used as an indicator of publication quality. For example, the National Library of Medicine relies on a panel of subject experts, the Literature Selection Technical Review Committee, to evaluate journals for indexing in the MEDLINE database.

When considering newly published journals, however, the library can only speculate, based on quality and content factors, whether a particular title will be picked up by a major index. The National Library of Medicine normally does not consider journals for indexing until they have been published for at least a year [24].

Bibliometric Indicators

Bibliometrics, or statistical bibliography, analyzes literature by numerically examining the publications of a discipline. Citation analysis reviews the references in a bibliography or database. These methods can be used to construct a profile of the literature or to help in selection. Analysis of the literature using statistical methods can aid not only in evaluating journals that have been published for some time, but in selecting journals to cover a subject area not previously or adequately supported by the library. Data can be used to identify journals with the greatest number of articles on a subject or that cover the greatest percentage of the literature—the core journals. The results of citation analysis for approximately 6,000 journals in the sciences are published by the Institute for Scientific Information (ISI) in *SCI Journal Citation Reports* [25]. These reports sort journals indexed by ISI into subject groups and rank them by various measures, including the number of articles published, the total number of times the journal was cited in a given year, and the impact factor (average number of current citations to articles published in the previous two years). Also available from ISI is a data set, *Journal Performance Indicators on Diskette*, which allows users to manipulate journal information, including the number of papers published and citation impact, within specific time periods from 1981-1994 [26].

Bibliometric data must be used cautiously as a selection tool [27-29]. The correlation between citations and journal use is not straightforward. Journals are used for news, current information, policy discussions and clinical case reporting, as well as for research. Citations are only one indicator of value. Articles may be cited for multiple reasons and not necessarily to indicate useful research or clinical content. The ease with which bibliographic data can be downloaded from online or CD-ROM databases and transferred to spreadsheet or database management programs makes it practical for libraries to apply bibliometric techniques for their unique needs [30]. Bibliometric methods have been used to create core lists of journals in various specialized fields, such as socioeconomics [31], tropical medicine [32], and family practice [33].

Physical Quality

Not all countries have equal access to high-quality paper and printing, but the physical characteristics of a sample issue can be important in making a decision to subscribe to a journal.

Illustrations

The importance of illustrative material will vary according to a journal's subject content. Where reproduction of radiographs, photographs, or other images is critical to the content, clarity and definition are essential. In some fields, use of color is important. If the quality of the illustrations is questionable, the potential users of the journal are a good source of advice.

Paper and Binding

Acid-free paper is becoming more common and is relevant primarily to historical preservation. While use of acid-free paper is an important goal for the profession to request of publishers and printers, it is rarely a factor that enters into a library's decision to subscribe to a publication. The users' information needs should always be the driving force. More important in the short run is whether the issues are bound so that the pages stay together.

Users Need

Current needs should guide selection of journals for the local collection. Few major research libraries now have a mission that includes responsibility for preserving in depth the record of current knowledge and anticipating the needs of tomorrow's scholars. For most health sciences libraries patient care and current research needs will drive the decisions about what to include in library collections.

One indicator of need is the number of requests made to obtain copies of articles through interlibrary loan or document delivery services. In addition, libraries that have department representatives who serve as advisors on the collection should make use of this link to obtain information regarding current needs. While any individual representative may be more or less able to reflect all department needs and will certainly tend to emphasize his or her own interests, these representatives should offer a window on institutional priorities, at least at the department level. Journals that are sponsored by a professional society are likely to be known to local members of that society, who may then request that the library subscribe.

Local Availability

Local availability may be another factor to consider before subscribing to a journal. If the library doesn't own the title, it should ascertain how quickly and easily articles can be obtained. If the health sciences library is on a main university campus and the journal is available at another library on campus, that is usually sufficient, with a few exceptions for intensely used publications. A daily campus delivery system or routine transmission by fax will enable efficient collection sharing. As budgets shrink, duplication within campuses tends to be minimized in favor of maintaining a larger number of titles. Libraries that belong to a regional network or consortium may wish to coordinate their collections, duplicating only the heavily used materials and encouraging acquisition of unique materials that are needed by the region or group but at a level that can be handled by a single copy. As document delivery equipment that digitizes images and reproduces graphics and color at original quality becomes more common, reliance on remote collections or commercial document delivery services is becoming increasingly acceptable.

Cost

Journal prices have been a very visible problem for the past two decades, engendering much emotional discussion regarding publishers' pricing policies, institutional support for library budgets, intellectual property rights, and responsibility for disseminating scientific scholarship. Amid the swirling debate and attempts to deal with the issues on a broad scale, individual selection decisions must still be made. Cost will usually be a factor in deciding whether to subscribe to a title. If there are multiple journals in the same field, a judgment must be made whether they are equivalent in content value. If one is significantly more expensive, it should provide sufficient added value for the cost, such as more articles, more authoritative articles, better illustrations, and probably most critical— important new information that will not appear elsewhere. The judgment on benefit for cost may be difficult. Subject experts should be called upon for advice.

Electronic Journals

Electronic journals in the health sciences will require increasing attention by libraries. While many issues related to electronic publications in general are covered in Chapter 6, Selection: Electronic Resources, the electronic format for journals is treated here. Selection becomes more challenging as more factors must be considered than for print journals [34]. Information on availability of electronic journals is published by the Association of Research Libraries (ARL) in both print and electronic formats [35].

Electronic journals may be categorized by mode of access: remote access through a commercial vendor, or local access through CD-ROM, floppy disk, or other electronic format loaded on a library workstation or institutional network. Electronic journals may also be categorized by content: an electronic version of a print journal, such as *JAMA* or *New England Journal of Medicine,* or an exclusively electronic publication, such as the *Online Journal of Current Clinical Trials.* For discussion of selection factors for electronic journals, three combinations of these two groupings are considered.

Access to Electronic Versions of Print Journals

Full text versions of a growing number of medical journals are available online through database vendors. In 1992 one vendor, BRS, offered access to seventy-two current titles in clinical medicine. In 1996 Ovid Technologies offered forty-five biomedical journals. Because these are common, heavily used journals, few libraries are likely to consider relying on online access as a substitute for a print subscription. More often, the electronic version is useful to individuals who wish to see the full text of an article after identifying the citation from a database search. As access to electronic versions of journals widens and the number of titles available increases, providing users with copies produced from a central database may become cost effective. Ultimately, most users will have the necessary technology to receive, display, and print articles at their own workstations. Document delivery, coupled with journal contents services now offered by some vendors, is still primarily paper-based. The issues that electronic journals pose for libraries are not substantially different than those posed by print journals. However, there are additional factors. The following sets of questions may guide decision making.

Access

Can the user get to the information easily? How much time and expertise is needed to use the network and the database to locate and acquire copies of articles? Is the software interface truly user friendly? What equipment is needed for receipt of article copies if transmitted electronically? Can the user download or print the copy directly or are additional steps required for delivery?

Quality

Is the content complete? Is the journal reproduced cover to cover, or are some sections, such as letters or book reviews omitted? Does the electronic version include all the graphic images of the print version? How adequate is the copy quality of the transmitted document? How does the format differ from the print version?

Speed

How quickly is the content transmitted, both for viewing and for downloading or printing? Is additional equipment required for maximum transmission speed? What is the impact of other resources used on the same equipment?

Local Electronic Versions of Print Journals

As with remote access to electronic versions of print journals, content decisions are no different from selecting the print version, with several additional questions to answer.

User Interface

Is the software easy to use, both for novice and experienced users? How fast is it? What is the quality of images and graphics? Are there indexes or searching and browsing capabilities? Consider whether the electronic version offers unique features, such as interactive functions, attached compressed files for additional data, sound or animation, or specialized graphics.

Access

Can the user get to the electronic version as easily as to the print version? Will the electronic version be available only in the library, or will the user be able to access it from office, hospital, or home? Is special equipment required? Does the user have to go through several layers of menus or commands to reach the articles?

Equipment Requirements

Does the library have the computer capacity to load the files and maintain acceptable response times? What operating system is required and is it compatible with the locally used platform? Is the library positioned to maintain hardware and software support through new versions and possible system changes? Can the system accommodate an adequate number of simultaneous users? Is the display capability good?

Duplication

Electronic versions may be acquired as a space-saving measure in a small library, to substitute for the printed journal. If backfiles of journals are easily available on optical disc or other electronic format, a library might consider not retaining the older printed volumes. Decisions should be made carefully, taking into account the library's role in preserving the content permanently and the current state of technology. The archival properties of CD-ROM or optical disc storage have not been proven. Duplication in both formats will be expensive and is not likely to be justifiable on grounds of need.

Cost

Electronic versions of full text journals are in an evolutionary state; both the technology and the pricing structures are in flux. A library may be able to obtain a set of journals on CD-ROM through a publisher or vendor. Pricing methods may include leasing agreements, charges for individual use, and other factors. Both long- and short-term costs, including equipment and maintenance, must be carefully weighed against the benefits to the user.

Original Electronic Journals

Journals accessed remotely through telecommunications are likely to dominate the future of electronic publications. Now in its infancy, this format will become more prevalent. As it develops, numerous issues must be addressed by publishers, distributors, and libraries. Libraries may have differing roles: as originators of electronic publications for their institutions, as managers or coordinators, as trainers, as users, and as preservers.

Access

As with a print journal, the user may choose to access or subscribe to an electronic journal individually. The future role of libraries as a locus for access to resources only reached through telecommunications is less clear. The library may subscribe and make publications available from workstations within the library only, or also by access through an institutional network. Decisions have to made about how the publication is managed, what responsibility the library has for maintaining records, and what information should appear in the local catalog. The library's archival responsibilities must be defined. The same questions about equipment and user interface as have been raised regarding all electronic resources also apply. If the journal has multimedia features, the library will need to assess its capability for receiving and decompressing files and for downloading graphics and images to produce sound and display animated video.

Quality

An electronic journal for which there is no print counterpart should be judged in terms of content by the same criteria as printed journals. Assessments must be made about the publishers, the editors, and the authors. The process for editorial and peer review should be ascertained. Lag time for publication should be determined. Electronic publishing has the potential for greatly speeding the dissemination of articles, but this should be demonstrated before a decision is made. If illustrations are a significant element of the journal, the quality must be acceptable. Special features should be reviewed and evaluated.

Cost

Electronic access enables both the publisher and a library intermediary more alternatives for charging. It is possible to track use and therefore to charge by use, or by password, or by number of simultaneous users. When these factors come into play, the library also has an option of recovering costs directly from the user, if the library is paying for the subscription. Decisions are further complicated by any additional costs for equipment to access and print files.

Gifts

Reliance on gifts of journals must be considered with care [36]. For journals in heavy demand or central to the collection, donated copies should be avoided. However, gift copies of common heavily used journals may be welcomed to fill in for missing issues or replace tattered ones at the time a volume is bound. If the library can expand its coverage by adding a title that is somewhat peripheral to the core collection, but still useful, a donation could be considered.

If loyal library users offer their personal copies of journals—"to help out"—should the library accept? When the budget is reduced and journal subscriptions must be canceled, should the library solicit donated copies? The answer to both questions is a qualified "maybe." In most cases the library will not choose to rely on an individual's personal subscription, primarily because it is likely to be an erratic and unreliable source. Donors may subscribe to a journal because its contents are important to their work or they may receive it as a benefit of membership in an organization. If the donor wants to read the journal before turning it over to the library, there will be a lag time and generally an unpredictable one. It may be difficult or uncomfortable for the library to claim issues that haven't been received. A reasonable waiting period is likely to be longer with a donor than with a publisher or vendor. Meanwhile the library users are without the latest issue. At best, this is an awkward situation.

Some publishers with dual pricing practices for individuals and institutions, fearing libraries will turn to individuals to supply the library with their personal subscriptions, have taken measures to prevent this practice. By printing "not for library use" on the cover, they contend such use is illegal.

Gifts of subscriptions to nonmedical periodicals of general interest may be welcome and may be the best way to obtain a leisure reading collection without using institutional collection funds.

Review and Deselection

Once a decision has been made—often far in the past—to subscribe to a journal and an unbroken set of volumes graces the library shelves, reversing that decision and discontinuing the journal seems particularly painful. However good a library's budget may be and however adequate its space, regular and systematic review of journal subscriptions should be as integral to collection management as selection of new journals. And, of course, it is a rare library where the staff judge either the budget or space to be adequate.

As an institution grows and its mission shifts, research interests and clinical emphasis will also change. Except in the very few large research institutions with a broader purpose, the library's local collections will reflect the primary current needs. Periodic assessment of collections will measure how well, within the institution's resources, the library is meeting those needs. Criteria for evaluating the collection and methods of assessment are covered more thoroughly in Chapter 9, Collection Assessment.

Whatever method is selected, the process should include some means of involving the library's primary user groups.

Ongoing Review

The method and frequency of reviewing journal subscriptions may depend on the size of the collection and the degree of flexibility in the budget. Libraries with static and inflexible budgets may follow a policy of only adding new titles when existing subscriptions of equivalent monetary value are canceled. Even when this is the case, the review and decision process should be systematic rather than a series of isolated decisions. A ranked list of potential candidates for deselection can be used for comparison when evaluating new titles.

A complete review of current subscriptions every two to three years is a reasonable standard. Guidelines for such a review appear in Chapter 9, Collection Assessment. For comprehensive biomedical collections, the evaluation may be undertaken in stages over time, evaluating several disciplines in each review period with the result that the entire collection will be examined within the specified time frame. This process spaces the effort and makes it easier to involve staff and users in the review.

The purpose of ongoing regular evaluation of subscriptions is to winnow out those titles that are no longer needed or are judged to be of lower quality than other publications covering the same field. The desired result is a collection of the highest quality journals that answers most needs for current information. Those libraries with a mission of providing a broad historical record of knowledge and practice and supporting a more diverse population of users will not focus quite so narrowly on current interests.

Single Purpose Evaluation

In times of financial crisis due to unexpected price increases, budget cuts, or reordered priorities, a more elaborate and stringent review process may be required, with a specific dollar goal to be achieved. The purpose is more focused and the target more obvious, but the process is essentially the same. Some libraries have described their review process [37-39].

And what of the broken runs of journals? The unbroken set should not become a sacred cow. If needs and resources change and the once-canceled journal is reinstated, no one should sigh over the gaps. While less tidy, the gaps can be easily recorded in most automated library systems, making it possible both to identify what the library has on hand and in finding another library that does have the needed volume and from which an article can be obtained. Fast delivery of articles makes these gaps less serious for the local user and as the gap recedes into the past the absent volumes will be less and less missed.

Book Selection

Book selection may take place on a macro level through approval plans or standing orders for series, or on a micro level through title-by-title selection. Many health sciences libraries use a combination of both approaches. Regardless of the method used for selecting, the primary consideration must be that the books acquired fit the collection development policy and fill a real need.

The Process

In Chapter 2, models for concentrating or distributing book selection responsibilities were reviewed. In libraries where some of the selection activities are delegated to someone other than the collections manager or library director, the responsibilities should be formally agreed upon and the flow of information and decisions clearly delineated. When most of the book selecting is distributed among several persons, a manual describing both the responsibilities and the process is useful. As a reference source for selectors and a training tool for new staff, the value of a manual lies in promoting consistency and thoroughness in carrying out the functions. By documenting expectations, the manual can also assist a manager with performance reviews.

In a small library there will be little confusion regarding who has what responsibility related to selection. As staff size increases, however, the need for a defined process increases. Procedures will need to document how publishers' announcements are handled, who sees them, how they are divided, for instance by subject, and how they are marked for follow up. If book reviews in medical or library journals are used as sources by selectors, a routing process should be established. A method for transmitting order information from the selector to the individual responsible for ordering needs to be agreed upon, including the types of notations or symbols to be used. If selections are reviewed by the collection manager or library director before ordering, a schedule or pattern for review will encourage a predictable workflow. If individual selectors review interlibrary loan requests, there must be a mechanism for receiving that information. Reports of lost books or heavy use of individual books are useful to selectors for decisions about replacements or added copies, but the information will only be transmitted if it is built into a routine. While these matters may seem trivial, attention to clearly defining the flow of information will pay off in increased effectiveness and more cooperative relationships among staff.

The link between selection activity and the collection budget must also be established. If individual selectors have any fund management responsibilities, such as working with subject-specific allocations or funds for specialized collections, reports on expenditures, encumbrances, and balances will be needed on a timely basis. Even if book selection is distributed without budget responsibilities, periodic reports regarding the status of the budget should be distributed. If selectors need to respond to budget conditions by speeding up or slowing down the number of recommendations they make, they should be thoroughly informed and given as much forewarning as possible. When establishing workflow patterns, all those with a role in the process should keep in mind the goal—to offer the best service to the user. Having materials available at the time they are needed should be the desired end that drives the process, not just an accidental byproduct of procedures that are convenient for staff.

Applying Collection Policy and Selection Criteria

Specific criteria for book selection are covered in Chapter 4, and they include the following: subject scope in relation to collection policy, content quality, audience, currency, technical quality of the book, local availability, and cost.

In those libraries that rely substantially on approval plans the selector has an opportunity to make judgments by examining the actual book. Many of these criteria can be assessed even when direct examination is not possible. Atkinson has described a model of the mental process by which individual decisions are made [40]. In what he calls the "syntagmatic context," the selector makes assumptions about content and quality from elements in the citation, such as publisher, place, date, length, author, title. In the "supplemental context," this information may be supplemented by additional data, such as subject classification, presence on a core list, a book review, or examining a copy on approval. In the "context of resolution" the selector uses all the gathered information about the item and considers it in relation to what the selector knows about the collection (historical precedence), the subject, and the library's clientele. A balance among these three contexts must be achieved in making selection decisions.

Historical Precedence

Existing collection strengths may drive some selection decisions. If a library has over the years developed a strong collection in a specialized area to meet the information needs of a segment of the user group, and if it has gained recognition as a comprehensive source in that field, it may continue adding materials to the collection at a level not required by current user needs. The library's collection policy should guide decisions about the depth of collecting; the library's budget will determine the degree to which the policy can be carried out. Selectors and collection managers should be familiar both with the existing collections and with the policy statements.

Subject Knowledge

The importance of understanding subject areas for which materials are selected has been discussed in some detail in Chapter 3, Education and Training for Collection Development. In biomedicine and related health care fields, scientific advances and changes in practice occur continually and rapidly. The selector must be alert to new methods, new technology, new diseases, new cures, new drugs, new policies, new issues, and constantly changing terminology. Publishers are quick to capitalize on changing interests and new developments. Selectors need to be able to judge critically the value of yet another slim expensive volume in a very specialized field. Familiarity with authors, publishers, and other publications in the field is essential for making discriminating choices.

User Needs

Continually updated knowledge of research programs, curriculum changes, and specialized clinical services will greatly aid selectors in choosing books for the collection. Sources are news publications from the institution, descriptions of grant awards, faculty activities and publications, even the local news media. Attendance at lectures or seminars will familiarize selectors with current research interests. Attendance at grand rounds or continuing education programs may highlight clinical topics of current concern. Participation on professional school or hospital committees can provide valuable insights as program emphases change or new programs are planned. In academic settings, a librarian should, if possible, be a member of the curriculum committee, or should at least receive copies of committee minutes and reports. This is one of the best ways to find out about new courses or shifts in how courses are taught. The impact on the library collections of both types of change should be assessed. New courses may require greater depth in both book and journal collections. A change in teaching method from a lecture format to more problem-centered or case-based independent learning may place greater demands on library materials. Methods for assessing the existing collection to incorporate a new program responsibility and to determine the degree to which the library can support a proposed program are described in Chapter 9.

Keeping a profile of research or clinical interests may be useful, particularly in academic health sciences libraries with a large and diverse clientele. Some universities maintain campus-wide directories, based on active research grants. With a database management system, developing a profile using Medical Subject Headings (MeSH) or other appropriate terminology can be relatively easy [41]. Another approach is to rely on citation information from external sources, such as the Institute for Scientific Information (ISI) [42]. The challenge is to collect the information systematically and maintain current profiles [43].

Sources of Information

Published Sources

New publications from major medical and scientific publishers are easy to identify. Publishers' advertisements and catalogs, cataloging records from the National Library of Medicine or other libraries' acquisitions lists, and book reviews in biomedical or library journals are commonly used sources. The challenge is to obtain the information as quickly as possible, with the least effort, avoiding redundancy but missing little. The number of sources used will depend on how comprehensive or, conversely, how selective the collection is. The depth of collecting for different topics within a library may vary; the sources used to identify materials will also vary accordingly. A hospital library serving clinical services and residency programs will emphasize standard texts covering major specialties. Publishers' or vendors' announcements will alert librarians to new editions of existing works [44]. For entirely new works, the library with a limited collection may wish to wait for a review to appear in journals such as *JAMA, New England Journal of Medicine, Annals of Internal Medicine, American Journal of Nursing,* or other specialty journals [45]. *Doody's Health Sciences Book Review Journal,* started in October 1993, publishes descriptive information about content [46]. Approximately 60% of listings include signed expert opinions written by health professionals, primarily affiliated with academic medical centers in Illinois.

User Recommendations

Recommendations from the library's users should always be seriously considered. This does not mean that every item recommended by a user is purchased. Several questions should be asked. How well does the book fit into the scope of the collection? How likely are others to use it? What is the projected cost per use? The same criteria should be applied to items requested by a user as to those selected by the library. The advantage of a user-generated request is knowing that it will be used by at least one person. The library must balance the value of anticipating needs and having materials on the shelves at the time someone wants it against the likelihood that no one will want it and therefore the costs of purchasing, cataloging, and shelfspace are wasted. It is not always easy to apply the "just in time" versus "just in case" theories, when for some people and in some situations "just in time" means having the item available when the information need arises, that is, "now." Until the processes for acquiring and physically delivering materials by purchase or interlibrary borrowing can be altered to eliminate the considerable time barrier, especially for books, health sciences libraries must attempt to anticipate their users' needs. Recommendations from users for materials not yet published can be a window onto these needs. Also, patterns of interlibrary borrowing may point out gaps in subject areas and suggest publications that should be acquired [47].

Approval Plans

Many health sciences libraries use approval plans to acquire books that match a defined profile. The plan itself is a selection tool. Crafting the profile to be used by the vendor in identifying which books to send on the plan is an act of selection. The profile should express the criteria in the library's collection policy, not only in terms of subject scope, but type of material, primary user groups, and other nonsubject parameters. If the library has a general policy of not acquiring conference proceedings or examination review books, then these types of publications should be excluded from the approval plan. A smaller library may wish the approval plan to cover only certain publishers or may restrict its profile to new editions of books on the Brandon/Hill list. (See Table 5-1.)

As the name denotes, an approval plan offers a second opportunity to select, after the books have been received. Two decisions must be made: 1) how closely to review books received through the approval plan, and 2) how thoroughly to monitor the plan's coverage of books that fall within its scope. The primary reason to use an approval plan is efficiency: to obtain core materials more quickly, avoid the process of placing individual orders, and reduce the time devoted to the selection effort [48].

While the library should periodically evaluate how well the plan succeeds in achieving the coverage it promises, the monitoring process should not be so thorough that it erases the benefit of having the plan. When returns are substantial the profile may need to be revised or clarified. Most vendors are quite flexible in accommodating the library's needs, understanding that purchasing, especially in small libraries, may be abruptly curtailed by budget restraints. Monitoring the reasons for return (out of scope, too elementary, already have enough on this topic, etc.) can aid both the vendor and the library in deciding if the profile needs to be adjusted. If the profile is so nonspecific or the vendor so unreliable that the work of selection must be essentially duplicated, then the plan is probably not achieving its goal.

Core Lists

Health sciences libraries with clinical collections, especially those serving hospitals, will find core lists especially useful for selection of both books and journals. For libraries with severely limited budgets, a list of titles that have been carefully selected as the authoritative texts in medical or other health specialties can assist with difficult decisions. One of the most commonly used sources is the "Selected List of Books and Journals for Small Medical Libraries," compiled biannually by Alfred Brandon and Dorothy Hill and known familiarly as the "Brandon/Hill list." This list is published in the April issue of the *Bulletin of the Medical Library Association* in odd-numbered years. Another heavily used source is the "Library for Internists," published every three years in the *Annals of Internal Medicine*. The purpose of this listing is to aid small libraries in selecting materials and to suggest items for students and practitioners to purchase for their own personal libraries. Titles listed are the result of nominations solicited by the American College of Physicians from its members. Specialized lists of materials in allied health or other specialty fields may be used, both for initial selection or as a standard for evaluating an existing collection. (See Table 5-1.)

Selection of Special Types of Material

Selection criteria should relate not only to subject scope and level of scholarship, but to a variety of formats and types of content. The selector needs to give special attention to these materials. Historical collections are discussed separately in Chapter 7.

Documents

Government documents can be problematic to identify and acquire. If the health sciences library is associated with an institution that is a depository for U.S. government documents, acquisition of publications from major health agencies may be automatic. The health sciences library and the general academic library may choose to divide responsibility, with health agency documents housed in the health sciences library. As fewer government publications are issued in printed form, the library may need to devote more effort to providing access through locally acquired non-print formats or online databases. The *Monthly Catalog of United States Government Publications,* available in numerous formats, is the primary source for identifying individual publications [49]. With the rapidly expanding capabilities of the Internet, many government publications are readily available through communication servers for viewing or file transfer into the user's computer.

Dissertations

Most universities maintain archival collections of dissertations written for degrees conferred by the home institution. Typically these copies are centralized in a single collection, although they may be dispersed in subject-based libraries throughout the campus. The health sciences library may retain theses or dissertations in the biomedical sciences or health professions, such as nursing, public health, or pharmacy. Unless a library is attempting a comprehensive collection in a very specialized area, dissertations from other institutions will rarely be acquired. When requested by a user, they are generally borrowed from the originating institution or purchased by or for the individual requester.

Technical Reports

In some biomedical fields, such as biomedical engineering or aerospace medicine, technical reports may be as important as journal literature. Organizations such as the Institute of Electrical and Electronics Engineers (IEEE) or the National Aeronautics and Space Administration (NASA) issue report series that contain important information. If the institution has significant programs in areas such as biomedical engineering or space medicine, technical reports will be sought. Research collections should include technical report literature when applicable. As with government documents, a growing amount of report literature is available electronically.

Textbooks

Questions about collecting textbooks arise primarily in teaching institutions. How many medical, nursing, dentistry, pharmacy, or veterinary medicine textbooks should be acquired? How many copies of texts recommended by the faculty should be made available by the library? The library's role in the learning environment should be assessed and expectations clarified with the health professional schools before a policy regarding textbooks is established. The current trend is for fewer students to purchase textbooks because of cost, or because they rely on reprinted readings or class notes instead. Even fewer may read them, either their own or library copies [50]. Those who do read assigned material may turn to the library and expect copies to be available.

Textbook collections may be handled in one of several ways. Traditionally, assigned textbooks have been kept in closed reserve collections, for use within the library for limited periods of time, or possibly loaned overnight. As assigned readings often take the form of reprints or photocopies, demand for the physical book has in some cases diminished. Another approach is for the library to maintain a current core collection, with a variety of textbooks, openly accessible but for use in the library. This approach allows easier access and encourages use of multiple sources, for comparison and greater depth of information. A third method of making textbooks available is to integrate representative texts into the library's reference collection. Combining textbooks as reference material can add convenience for librarians who frequently consult such texts to answer queries. Whether interspersing textbooks with dictionaries, directories, and other information sources serves the needs of students could be questioned but has not been studied.

Regardless of how textbooks are managed in the library, some general guidelines will be needed as to how broadly to collect. Texts written by or recommended by current faculty in the institution are obvious choices. A selected number of standard texts from core lists will be expected. Specialty textbooks in fields of importance to the research programs or clinical services will also be needed.

Review Books

Programmed texts and examination review books pose additional questions for the selector. These types of materials should be addressed in the library's collection policy. Some libraries will choose not to acquire them, leaving these learning tools for the individual student to purchase. It can be argued that such materials do not represent knowledge as do textbooks, monographs, and journals. The counter argument is that they represent a means of learning, similar to computer-assisted learning programs or interactive media, and are therefore appropriate for the library to acquire. With the growth of computer-based teaching tools, the review book may fade away.

Leisure Reading

Many health sciences libraries cater at least minimally to the view that the health sciences library serves a social as well as a scholarly function. Not only is the library a place for study, research, and fact-finding, but it also serves as a haven away from the laboratory, clinic, office, and class-room—a place for temporary relief from the stress of patient care or barrage of facts to learn. Recognizing this function, the library may subscribe to a small number of local or national newspapers, current events magazines, and other light reading materials. The days of acquiring selected volumes of literature or subscriptions to a variety of magazines out of the library's collection budget have largely vanished. Most often, these small collections will be provided through donations, from staff, regular users, or benefactors.

Gifts

Gifts of books, like gifts of journals, frequently come to the library as a result of retirement, death, or simply a lack of office space in which to keep them. Unsolicited gifts are generally unwanted gifts, but may often be accepted, both for the public relations value (people often feel sentimental about their private collections) and because the collections may indeed contain valuable items. For large collections it is best to get a good description, obtain a list of contents from the donor, or in some cases examine the collection before accepting it. If the material is clearly unusable and the library has no good means of disposing of the collection, the best solution may be to gently explain to the donor why it doesn't match the library's current needs. Offering alternatives, if they are reasonable ones, may soften the blow. Quick screening will usually identify whether there are likely to be current materials that fit the scope of the collection or historical gems, suitable for those libraries that collect in depth or maintain historical collections.

To comply with Internal Revenue Service requirements, donors wishing to claim gifts to the library valued over $200 in a year for tax deductions should be encouraged to seek an appraisal. The library may not appraise potential gifts, nor under usual circumstances pay for the appraisals [51].

In offering gifts not needed by the library, or items withdrawn from the collection, to charitable organizations or agencies that distribute books and journals to needy countries, the library should be certain that the material falls within the scope of need and will be truly useful. There may be no benefit in sending substantially outdated clinical or scientific information.

Book sales or give-away tables can also be considered. Donors need to know that unneeded gifts may be disposed of in this manner. The library must also take into account staff costs associated with management, tax collection, or record keeping for book sales. Figures 5-3 and 5-4 include examples of gift policies.

Review and Discard

Even the most comprehensive collections need to be evaluated periodically and purged of materials no longer needed. Space is eventually a problem in every library and except for those few academic health sciences libraries that serve as historical repositories and centers for scholarship, retaining large numbers of outdated and unused books is a disservice to users by making the library more cumbersome to use and by including clinical information that is no longer accurate or applicable. In making decisions about what to keep and what to withdraw, the library should refer both to its mission and to its collection policy.

If the library's purpose is primarily to serve clinical and teaching needs, it will have little justification for maintaining a collection of earlier editions of texts and reference works. On the other hand, a library with a mission to support research or programs in the history of the health sciences might choose to maintain representative examples of earlier works, in order to understand the evolution of knowledge and practice, and the diffusion of ideas. Libraries serving substantial biomedical research programs will have greater need to retain specialized materials, especially if they continue to be used.

For the collection to reflect the library's policy, a plan for systematic review should be followed. Some decisions may be built in: if the policy is to keep only the latest two editions of standard textbooks, then removal of earlier editions can be automatic when a new edition is received. Multiple copies of earlier editions may also be systematically withdrawn. Weeding earlier works not only reduces clutter and space consumption, but also removes the incentive for students or laypersons to consult outdated material.

More elaborate review and weeding programs will be conducted less frequently. Collection evaluation may be viewed as applying the collection policy in reverse, with the addition of criteria such as history of use,

GIFTS TO THE LIBRARY

Since the founding of The New York Academy of Medicine, the Library collections have been enriched by generous gifts of books and other materials. The Library welcomes gifts of books that fall within the scope of its collecting activities and which support the Academy programs. Of particular interest are scholarly or rare items with research value that are in good physical condition. Materials which fall outside the Library's collection policy such as popular journals, unnecessary duplicates, unbound reprints, etc. are generally not accepted. Sets of relevant journals will be accepted if they are intact with original covers, advertisements, supplemental materials, etc.

POLICY : Gifts of materials are accepted by the Library with the understanding that upon receipt, the Academy becomes the owner of the materials. The Library reserves the right to determine their retention based on their suitability for the collection, location, cataloging treatment and other considerations related to their use or disposition. Only the Academy Librarian or his/her designees may accept books on behalf of the Library.

PROCEDURES : Anyone interested in donating materials should send a list of the materials to the Acquisitions Department, The New York Academy of Medicine Library, 2 East 103rd Street, New York, NY 10029-5293. The librarian will contact the donor and indicate whether or not the gift would be of value to the Library. Delivery to the Library is generally the donor's responsibility and the cost may be tax deductible.

APPRAISALS : Donors who wish an evaluation of their gifts for tax purposes are referred to the Internal Revenue Service Publication 561, Determining the Value of Donated Property, and Publication 526, Charitable Contributions. If the value of the gift exceeds $500, the donor must submit a list giving author, title, place, publisher and date of all items and must complete IRS Form 8283, Noncash Charitable Contributions. When the value exceeds $5,000, the donor must obtain an independent appraisal and the donor, appraiser and the Academy must all sign Form 8283. The donor is responsible for paying the cost of the appraisal, an expense that may be tax deductible. Because the Academy is considered an interested party in the transaction, the IRS will not approve an appraisal made or paid for by the Library.

GIFTS OF MONEY : Donations of funds to supplement the Library's acquisitions are welcomed. Information on making contributions to the Library, establishing an endowment and naming opportunities may be obtained from the Academy Librarian.

ACKNOWLEDGEMENTS : Appropriate acknowledgement of all gifts is made by the Library. Also, where appropriate, gift plates with the donor's name may be placed in the volumes.

Figure 5-3: Gift Policy (New York Academy of Medicine)

Dolph Briscoe, Jr. Library
The University of Texas Health Science Center at San Antonio

GIFT RECEIPT   Date_____

RECEIVED FROM _____

    Address   _____   Telephone _____

_____

SPECIAL INFORMATION _____

_____

_____

_____

Received by _____

Donors are listed in the Honor Roll of Contributors in the Library's annual report. Unless otherwise requested a copy of this receipt will generally be the only other acknowledgement of your gift. Please read below before signing.

                       Signature _____

INFORMATION FOR PROSPECTIVE DONORS

The Library actively seeks and welcomes gifts of books or other library materials, or money to support its programs.

All gifts are accepted subject to the approval of the UT Board of Regents. Donors should be aware that all gifts are accepted with the understanding that upon receipt the University becomes the owner of the material and, as such, reserves the right to determine retention, location, cataloging treatment, and other considerations relating to use or disposition.

The appraisal of a gift to the Library for income tax purposes is the responsibility of the donor since it is the donor, not the Library, who benefits from the tax deduction. To protect both its donors and itself, the Library, as an interested party, must not appraise gifts made to it. The Library will provide assistance as to sources of information for evaluation purposes and will suggest appropriate professional appraisers who might be consulted. Because of tax considerations, donors may wish to discuss prospective donations and appraisals with their attorneys.

Transportation of gift collections generally should be arranged by the donor. Deliveries should be scheduled with the Library in advance to arrive between 8 a.m. and 5 p.m., Monday through Friday. If a list of items will be needed, the donor should prepare the list before delivering the gift to the Library.

Appropriate acknowledgement of all gifts is made by the Library. In the case of memorial gifts and endowments, a special book plate is placed in each volume added.

Questions on gifts should be directed to the Assistant Library Director for Collection Development, Dolph Briscoe, Jr. Library, The University of Texas Health Science Center at San Antonio, 7703 Floyd Curl Drive, San Antonio, Texas 78284-7940. (512) 567-2400.

Donor Copy   UTHSCSA Briscoe Library Form P5.6 (10/89)

Figure 5-4: Gift Receipt and Gift Information Form (University of Texas Health Science Center at San Antonio)

information which was not known or predictable at the time of initial selection. Techniques for evaluating collections are addressed in detail in Chapter 9.

References

1. New journals review. Nature 1995 Sep 21; 377 (6546): 259-72.
2. JAMA: Journal of the American Medical Association. Weekly. Chicago: American Medical Association.
3. Serials Review. Quarterly. Ann Arbor, MI: Pierian Press.
4. The NLM Technical Bulletin. Bimonthly. Bethesda, MD: National Library of Medicine.
5. Current Contents. Weekly. Philadelphia: Institute for Scientific Information. Sections on Agriculture, Biology & Environmental Sciences; Clinical Medicine; Engineering, Technology & Applied Sciences; Life Sciences; Physical, Chemical & Earth Sciences; Social & Behavioral Sciences.
6. Colaianni LA. Peer review in journals indexed in Index Medicus. JAMA 1994 Jul 13; 72(2):156-8.
7. Garfunkel JM, Ulshen MH, Hamorck HJ, et al. Effect of institutional prestige on reviewers' recommendations and editorial decisions. JAMA 1994 Jul 13; 272(2):137-8.
8. Oxman AD, Sackett DL, Guyatt GH. For the Evidence-Based Working Group. Users' guides to the medical literature, I: How to get started. JAMA 1993 Nov 3; 270(17): 2093-5.
9. Guyatt GH, Sackett DL, Cook DJ. For the Evidence-Based Medicine Working Group. Users' guide to the medical literature, II: How to use an article about therapy or prevention, A: Are the results of the study valid? JAMA 1993 Dec 1; 270(21): 2598-601.
10. Guyatt GH, Sackett DL, Cook DJ. For the Evidence-Based Medicine Working Group. Users' guide to the medical literature, II: How to use an article about therapy or prevention, B: What were the results and will they help me in caring for my patients? JAMA 1994 Jan 5; 271(1): 59-63.
11. Jaeschke R, Guyatt G, Sackett DL. For the Evidence-Based Medicine Working Group. Users' guides to the medical literature, III: How to use an article about a diagnostic test, A: Are the results of the study valid? JAMA 1994 Feb 21; 271(5): 389-91.
12. Jaeschke R, Guyatt GH, Sackett DL. For the Evidence-Based Medicine Working Group. Users' guides to the medical literature, III: How to use an article about a diagnostic test. B: What are the results and will they help me in caring for my patients? JAMA 1994 Mar 2; 271(9): 703-7.
13. Levine M, Walter S, Lee H, Haines T, et al. For the Evidence-Based Medicine Working Group. Users' guides to the medical literature, IV: How to use an article about harm. JAMA 1994 May 25; 271 (20): 1615-9.
14. Larpacis A, Wells G, Richardson WS, et al. For the Evidence-Based Medicine Working Group. Users' guides to the medical literature, V: How to use an article about prognosis. JAMA 1994 Jul 20; 272(3): 234-7.
15. Oxman AD, Cook J, Guyatt GH. For the Evidence-Based Medicine Working Group. Users' guides to the medical literature, VI: How to use an overview. JAMA 1994 Nov 2; 272(17): 1367-71.
16. Haynes RB. Loose connections between peer-review clinical journals and clinical practice. Ann Intern Med 1990 Nov 1; 113(9): 724-8.

17. Haynes RB, Mulrow CD, Huth EJ, et al. More informative abstracts revisited. Ann Intern Med 1990 Jul 1; 113(1):69-76.

18. Hallmark J. Scientists' access and retrieval of references cited in their recent journal articles. Coll Res Libr 1994 May; 55(3): 199-209.

19. Ulrich's International Periodicals Directory. Annual. New Providence, NJ: RR Bowker.

20. SERLINE database [online]. Bethesda, MD: National Library of Medicine.

21. The serials directory : an international reference book. Annual. Birmingham, AL : EBSCO.

22. Eldredge JD. Accuracy of indexing coverage information as reported by serials sources. Bull Med Libr Assoc 1993 Oct; 81(4):364-70.

23. List of Serials Indexed for Online Users. Annual. Bethesda, MD: National Library of Medicine.

24. National Library of Medicine. Fact sheet. Journal selection for Index Medicus/MEDLINE. July 1991.

25. SCI Journal Citation Reports (microfiche, with printed guide). Annual. Philadelphia: Institute for Scientific Information.

26. Small H. Journal performance indicators on diskette: a window on the big picture. Curr Contents 1995 Sep 11; no. 37:3-7.

27. Bensman SJ. Journal collection management as a cumulative advantage process. Coll Res Libr 1985 Jan; 46(1):13-29.

28. Pan E. Journal citation as a predictor of journal usage in libraries. Coll Manage 1978 Spring; 2(1):29-38.

29. Stankus T, Rice B. Handle with care: use and citation data for science journal management. Coll Manage 1982 Spring/Summer; 4(1/2):95-110.

30. Burnham JF, Shearer BS, Wall JC. Combining new technologies for effective collection development: a bibliometric study using CD-ROM and a database management program. Bull Med Libr Assoc 1992 Apr; 80(2):150-6.

31. Austin T. Socioeconomic resources in medicine: review of the literature. Bull Med Libr Assoc 1984 Jul; 72(3):251-255.

32. Roelants G. Citation analysis in the field of tropical medicine. Ann Soc Belg Med Trop 1987 Dec; 67(4):315-8.

33. Sneiderman CA. Keeping up with the literature of family practice: a bibliometric approach. Fam Prac Res J 1983 Fall; 3(1):17-23.

34. Grochmal HM. Selecting electronic journals. Coll Res Libr News 1995 Oct;56(9): 632-54.

35. Directory of electronic journals, newsletters, and academic discussion lists. 5th ed. Washington, DC: Association of Research Libraries, May 1995.

36. Grefsheim SF, Bader SA, Meredith PA. Personal/departmental journal subscription: panacea or pandora for a library's journal collection? Bull Med Libr Assoc 1984 Apr 72(2):208-9.

37. Walter PL. Doing the unthinkable: canceling journals in a research library. Serials Libr 1990; 18(1/2):141-53.

38. Spang L. Reconciling rising serial costs, the serials budget, and reference needs in a medical library serials retrenchment program: a methodology. Med Ref Serv Quart 1995 Spring;14(1):33-44.

39. Metz P. Thirteen steps to avoiding bad luck in a serials cancellation project. J Acad Libr 1992 May;18(2):76-82.

40. Atkinson RW. The citation as intertext: toward a theory of the selection process. Libr Res Tech Serv 1984 Apr/Jun; 28(2):109-19.

41. Medical Subject Headings. Annual. Bethesda MD: National Library of Medicine.

42. Law DT. Innovative use of in-house current awareness profiles as a guide for collection development in a pharmaceutical library. Coll Res Libr News 1989 May; 50(5):372-4.

43. Richardson JM. Faculty research profile created for use in a university library. J Acad Libr 1990 Jul; 16(3):154-7.

44. A Major Report. Quarterly: Dallas: Majors Scientific Books.

45. Books of the year. Amer J Nurs 1994 Jan; 94(1):62, 64-70.

46. Doody's Health Sciences Book Review Journal. Quarterly. Oak Park, IL: Doody Publishing.

47. Byrd GD, Thomas DA, Hughes KE. Collection development using interlibrary loan borrowing and acquisitions statistics. Bull Med Libr Assoc 1982 Jan; 70(1): 1-9.

48. Hulbert LA, Curry DS. Evaluation of an approval plan. Coll Res Libr 1978 Nov; 39(6):485-91.

49. Monthly catalog of United States Government publications. Monthly. Washington, DC: Superintendent of Documents.

50. Taylor CR. Great expectations: the reading habits of year II medical students. New Engl J Med 1992 May 21; 326(21):1436-40.

51. Ash L. Appraisals of library collections and gift to libraries. In: Encyclopedia of library and information science, v.39, Suppl. 4. New York: Dekker, 1985:45-8.

6

Selection: Electronic Resources

"Science and technology multiply around us. To an increasing extent they dictate the languages in which we speak and think. Either we use those languages, or we remain mute."

J.G. Ballard

Many health sciences libraries have microcomputer centers or areas where workstations are concentrated in order to facilitate software distribution, user assistance, and instruction. However, access to electronic resources is often not restricted to special settings. This chapter treats collection development for electronic resources in general, irrespective of the site from which they are used. While selection decisions parallel those for print materials in many ways, electronic formats are treated in a separate discussion because their unique characteristics introduce additional factors to collection decision making and because these formats can affect information delivery, budgeting, equipment, and staffing in profound ways.

Electronic resources play an essential role in every health sciences library, whether it is a microcomputer-based catalog and telecommunications to a vendor-managed MEDLINE database, or includes CD-ROM databases, computer-assisted educational software, and a locally mounted subset of MEDLINE. These resources are usually expensive, often more expensive than their printed counterparts, if such exist. Pricing may reflect research and development costs for the developers. As computer-based information consumes a greater proportion of a library's budget, a correspondingly greater degree of care should be taken in making decisions regarding what the library will provide for its users. Both policy and procedures need to be defined. The Association for Library Collections and Technical Services

(ALCTS) has published a useful *Guide to Selecting and Acquiring CD-ROMs, Software, and Other Electronic Publications* [1].

Collection Policy

As knowledge-based computer programs in clinical medicine and other health care disciplines are improved and gain wider acceptance, they appear more commonly as library resources, especially if they can be consulted through remote access from offices or clinical care sites. As with print material, selection of computer software for use by students, hospital staff, faculty, clinicians, or researchers should be guided by the library's collection policy. Examples of policies for electronic datafiles and computer software can be found in the Medical Library Association's DocKit on Collection Policies [2]. The policy should address the criteria by which these resources are chosen. Scope, depth, and audience will define the boundaries.

Several types of software may be acquired by health sciences libraries:

> bibliographic
> full text: books, journals
> numeric or factual databases
> clinical assist programs for diagnosis or treatment decisions
> educational software, for example:
>> computer-assisted instruction packages
>> simulations of laboratory experiments, patient interviews
>> study guides and tests
> applications software, for example:
>> word processing
>> analytical or statistical packages
>> file management
>> telecommunications
> administrative functions or staff support

The following criteria illustrate the factors taken into account in the decision making process.

Scope

The primary criterion should be whether the resource fits the subject scope of the library. As with print materials, the subject focus will be primarily in health sciences disciplines. If the subject is peripheral to the library's core collecting responsibilities, this may be grounds to turn down a user's request or to seek extra budgetary funding.

Depth

The intensity of collecting in a discipline may dictate how many resources the library will acquire, or the degree of specialization needed. For example, if the neurosciences are not an area of intense collecting, then a library may not acquire the *Neurosciences Citation Index* database, especially if it already provides the more general *Science Citation Index.*

Audience

Perhaps a more critical question than for any other format is whose needs the library intends to serve with computer software. If the library's clientele includes health professional students, relevant resources will differ depending on whether the library supports the entire educational program or only the clinical training. In medical school settings, resources directly related to the curriculum will be the most commonly acquired software. The library should be cautious about acquiring programs that the students are not actually required to use for their coursework or patient care assignments. Schools that use a problem-based approach or emphasize self-directed learning may encourage students to use a wide array of resources. In schools with a more traditional curriculum, students have little time at their disposal and rarely turn to supplemental materials [3]. As with audiovisual materials, computer-based resources for student use should usually be selected with advice and recommendation from faculty or potential users.

For practitioners the library may consider specialized diagnostic assist software, electronic reference texts, treatment protocols, emergency treatment information, or drug resources.

If basic research is supported by the library, then the resources that will contribute to the research effectiveness of the institutions must be considered. Access to resources such as genetic databases, citation indexes, and electronic journals may be appropriate.

Selection Principles

Each library will need to establish a set of criteria to assist in making individual selections of electronic resources. The first decision should be whether the resource serves the mission of the library and fits the scope and depth defined in the collection policy. It should meet information needs of the library's users. Secondly, specific criteria should address the content, the user interface and retrieval software, the format, and the hardware and software required by the resource. These criteria may be applied as appropriate for the particular type of resource. Careful investigation and evaluation of the cost-effectiveness of different formats should precede any decisions. An information policy both for the library and for the institution will help guide these decisions.

Selection of resources in formats that have not been integrated into the library's collections, operations, processes, or services will require involvement of staff throughout the library, including those with responsibilities for collection development, user assistance, ordering, cataloging, and computer system support. Demas has suggested forming an electronic resources council as a "cross-functional forum for reviewing and approving selection of electronic resources that have not yet been fully mainstreamed" [4] to assess the impact of proposed new resources and to coordinate functions among library units.

Selection Criteria: Content

Many of the elements by which content scope and quality are judged will be the same regardless of format: print, electronic, or other media.

Quality

As with print materials and audiovisual media, computer programs with health sciences content must be judged on the quality of the material presented. Criteria include authoritativeness of the content, expertise of the authors, reputation of the producer, and comprehensiveness of the information. If illustrative material is important, quality of the images will be a critical factor. The use to which programs will be put will influence which factors are considered most heavily in choosing software programs. Computer-based diagnostic systems are used by physicians as a form of consultation or to produce lists of potential diagnoses. These programs must be judged carefully and should always be reviewed by the clinicians who may utilize them. Performance measures, such as the proportion of correct answers, comprehensiveness of the database, and relevance of retrieved possible diagnoses may differ among programs [5].

Currency

If the software is designed to assist with diagnostic or treatment decisions, regular updates should be provided. Some software programs, e.g. *Quick Medical Reference*—*QMR*, have a mechanism whereby earlier versions are inactivated after a specified time period, based on the expected date for the next release.

Content Usefulness

If the software is intended for student use and is being used as a teaching tool, it should offer features that contribute to learning, such as interactive capabilities or testing. Most educational software should be responsive to user input—either in the form of answers to questions or entry of data.

Multimedia products offer limitless possibilities for professional education, clinical problem-solving, and continuing education. They enable the user to simultaneously hear and see the heart beating and view the electrocardiograph tracing; to hear and see a lecture or patient interview. Resources that combine text and images, sound and movement, and that give the user control over the order, speed, size, and level of detail of information will transform the world of textbook medicine.

Clinical-assist software should offer more than highly accurate, up-to-date knowledge. It should be able to show relationships and probabilities, based on user input that would be impossible or extremely laborious to achieve otherwise. As a memory extender it must verify known information or alert the user to relationships, such as drug interactions, of which the clinician may be unaware or has forgotten. Diagnostic-assist tools should suggest possibilities that are reasonable and useful for the practitioner.

Relationship to Print Publications

If the resource has a print counterpart, one should consider whether the content of the electronic version is enhanced by additional material, such as expanded coverage of journals, abstracts, full text, citations, or other data. Several factors will influence the library's decision to acquire both a print and electronic version, or electronic only. These factors may include convenience of access; amount of demand, especially if competing with other resources on a single workstation or small network; and need for permanent preservation. Increasingly, monographs are accompanied by data diskettes. Updates may be offered electronically through networks.

Selection Criteria: User Interface

Ease of Use

Some users will be willing to struggle with programs that are complicated or require some diligence to use effectively, especially if they have a flair for computers or if use of the software is an essential part of the curriculum. Many will be patient or persistent. However, busy practitioners are likely to be intolerant of software that cannot be used with ease. Commands or menus should be intuitive or at least very clear; time should not be squandered with excessive steps to retrieve information. Graphical user interfaces (GUI) are easier and more enjoyable for most users, but even these interfaces can become confusing if they are too cluttered with choices and there are so many pathways that the user becomes disoriented. Screen displays should be easily understood. Comparison studies can be useful. An example is the forum sponsored by the National Library of Medicine to evaluate the different CD-ROM formats for MEDLINE [6].

Software Functions

The search engine or other control functions should be powerful enough to support the resource. Response time should be snappy. For database programs, consider whether the search interface permits use of Boolean operators (and, or, not), truncation, and adjacency features, and whether searches or search strategies can be saved.

Printing and Downloading Capability

Depending on the institutional network and workstation configurations, the ability to print and download from electronic files can be problematic. It is wise to investigate the specific requirements for these essential features, both for in-library and remote users. No one is more unhappy than a user who has identified material that precisely meets an immediate need, only to find that it can't be printed. Most will also wish to be able to send results of searches to another address via electronic mail.

Duplication of Print Publications

When software duplicates to a large extent a print publication, such as a textbook, the library must determine whether the electronic version offers additional features that justify its purchase. Can the user search topics more easily or move from one concept to another using a hypertext or a similar application? Will the software reformat information and display it in unique ways? Can illustrative material be manipulated or animated? Can data be extracted and manipulated for individual use?

Compatibility with Other Resources

When there is a choice, there may be an advantage to selecting as many resources as possible from the same vendor to minimize the number of different interfaces a user must learn. When the institution has a single interface used to access multiple information sources, regardless of their source, users will be more facile in using the range of resources available. Use of a common interface instead of the interface developed for the product, however, may inhibit the user's ability to maximize the particular database because all features may not be available.

Documentation and Guides

The producer should provide documentation and guidance in use of the resource. An adequate number of manuals should be supplied and they should be easy to consult. If there are help screens for various functions of the program, they should be easily accessed and understandable. They should address the question the user is likely to have at the point in the program where the help feature is activated. The user should be able to easily return to the previous step. An 800 number for help may be an advantage, but its usefulness can be impaired by long response times. The technical support staff should be knowledgeable and helpful.

Selection Criteria: Format

One of the most vexing questions libraries face is the choice of format when multiple options exist. Does the library provide access to an index or other resource only in print, on standalone CD-ROM or CD-ROMs on a local area network, by tapes mounted on the local institutional network, or by various routes to a remote utility through a gateway? The library should consider the following factors in making these decisions.

Users

Consider the likely users: members of a single department, individuals throughout the institution, or students in a professional education program. If the resource is applicable to very few, the cost of the resource and all the support it will require may not be justified.

Expected Use

Consider the anticipated demand. The number and frequency of use of each user group will affect decisions, not only about acquiring the resource, but about licensing, multiple-access points, and user assistance.

Accessibility

Consider the users and where will they want to use the resource: in the hospital, from labs and offices, in the library or learning center, from remote clinical sites, or from home. Convenient access to network resources will increase the likelihood that individuals will use the resource.

Content

If a resource is available in different formats, consider how they differ in comprehensiveness or specialized content. Compare the interface and performance characteristics. Is the electronic format updated more or less frequently than the print format? Software may offer full text indexing that is not possible from a print version. Some may bundle several resources together, such as textbooks, dictionaries, or other reference works and journal articles.

Costs

Consider the anticipated cost per use. Ongoing producer or vendor charges for maintenance, upgrades, and required new versions must be factored into cost decisions. Equipment and system or network costs must be evaluated, as well as other support costs.

Equipment

Consider whether the resource is compatible with local systems. Changes or upgrades may be required. Users may or may not have necessary equipment and software to access the resource. Does the library possess the needed expertise to support the resource? Even if it does, the library must judge where to put staff time and effort.

Legal Issues

Consider whether site or multiuser licenses are available. If restrictions apply to making backup copies, downloading, and printing the library needs to understand this and determine its impact on the local environment and anticipated use. If the publisher imposes restrictions that would inhibit the expected use, the library should attempt to negotiate a change or decide not to acquire the program.

General recommendations are very difficult to make. Each environment must be assessed in terms of its resources, users, needs, and opportunities to participate in shared systems. In a large institution it may be cost-effective to acquire and manage subsets of heavily used databases, such as MEDLINE. These may be part of a campus-wide , multicampus, or even state-wide system. On the other hand, a CD-ROM version may be the best choice for smaller libraries without network capabilities. Boss has suggested a method for cost analysis to guide decisions [7].

Selection Criteria: Hardware, Software, and Space Requirements

Designing microcomputer facilities within libraries is a sufficiently large topic to justify its own book, which fortunately has already been written. Hannigan and Brown discuss in detail considerations for equipment and space [8]. What is appropriate to note here is that the special needs for access to computer-based resources impose another significant set of questions to consider when building collections.

Space

A decision to acquire computer-based resources assumes the library has facilities for using them. One consideration in making decisions is whether the facilities are conducive to the type of use that will be made of them. Materials that are consulted quickly or do not require intense concentration may be used on workstations in busy open areas. If assistance is likely to be needed, workstations should be situated where help is easily available. Some individuals can work in a crowded, noisy environment. Others find it difficult and work more effectively where there are fewer distractions. The library should assess the needs of all its user groups when determining how to place workstations within the library and, in selecting electronic resources, consider whether they can be used effectively in the available setting.

Workstation Configuration

The library's networking capability needs to be considered. Do users have remote access to the network from outside the library? If all resources are on a network server, the library will need staff to manage the network resources effectively. Workstations dedicated to single resources should generally be avoided, except as needed to preserve constant access to the most heavily used resources, such as MEDLINE or the library's catalog. If the library has numerous resources requiring manipulation of CD-ROMs or diskettes, how convenient is access? There should be an adequate number of workstations for effective use of computer-based information resources. Resources that require proprietary hardware should be avoided if there are reasonable alternatives. Technology changes too rapidly to justify purchase of single-purpose dedicated equipment under most circumstances.

Compatibility

Consider whether the computer-based resource being evaluated is compatible with existing equipment. Memory must be sufficient and the machine fast enough for the type of content, such as images. The new software must be evaluated to assure that it won't conflict with any other resources on the same equipment, by disabling programs or degrading response time.

Additional Software

Determine whether the resource requires specific software, such as an operating system or database loader. Audio and video will require additional components. The existing hardware must be adequate to accommodate the required software or the library will need to budget for new or upgraded equipment. Staff expertise must be available to install and maintain it.

Licensing Agreements and Copyright Restrictions

Cramer has suggested several actions libraries should take when faced with license agreements for electronic products [9]:

1. Determine what you are going to do with the product prior to purchase or renewal.
2. Build a relationship with your legal staff.
3. Establish a contact with the vendor to answer questions.
4. Obtain a copy of the license agreement as part of selection process.
5. Understand local definitions of user, site, etc.
6. Be clear about deviations from the standard license agreement.
7. Spell out local requirements to vendor.
8. Be prepared to monitor use for compliance.

In some cases, especially for subscriptions to databases, the library does not own the software and if it discontinues the subscription must return the disks already received. Restrictions on access and use may also pertain and should be reviewed carefully prior to purchase.

If purchasing an electronic resource for which there is a corresponding printed product, any requirement to continue subscribing to the print version should be weighed against total costs and expected use for both formats. Some licensing agreements restrict use of databases to certain classes of users, such as students. If restrictions limit the usefulness of a resource significantly and acceptable modifications cannot be negotiated, the library may decide to forgo acquiring it.

Copyright guidelines for electronic formats are somewhat murky, but libraries should follow reasonable practices to protect software from abuse by prohibiting unauthorized copying and making information available to users. The library should prevent, to the degree possible, illegal downloading and copying of databases and full text files.

Policies on Applications Software

Some health sciences libraries have a role in providing tools that help their clientele manipulate information or accomplish tasks. Individual health professionals, especially faculty and researchers, will usually have computer resources available in their own offices and labs, and if they work at home, they are likely to have similar access to word processing and other general use software. They may expect the same resources when they escape to the library to work. Students, who depend more heavily on on-site use of the library, may also need access to applications software that, although not a medical resource, will nonetheless assist them in their studies. As personal computers have become more compact and convenient, users will more routinely bring their own computers with them. However, the library will likely continue to have a role in providing software applications through library-based network resources to which users can link from their own computers.

The library should have a policy on whether it acquires general purpose software in addition to subject-related resources. Once acquired, the library must then decide whether these types of software are considered part of the collection, that is, whether they are funded from the collection budget.

Word Processing

Although clearly not an information resource itself, word processing can facilitate notetaking, downloading information from other electronic resources, and writing papers or case reports.

File Management

Software that allows users to organize, format, and search references in their own bibliographies or assists with reprint file management may have a justifiable place in the library. Searches conducted by the user in the library may be downloaded and formatted for personal use. Library staff may have instructional programs that demonstrate how to use such software for better management of individual information files. Having the software and documentation available in the library for public use will complement the educational programs and encourage practice and continued use.

In selecting which program to acquire, compatibility with other resources such as journal contents services (online or locally managed files) or databases may be a factor. Whenever possible, users should be able to download or transfer references from searches into their own files with the least effort and without needing to reformat.

Authoring Software

Health sciences libraries that serve medical or other health professional schools may consider making available software that assists faculty in developing computer-assisted learning programs. Opportunities to use simulation software, hypertext programs, and other types of authoring programs may stimulate faculty to develop innovative approaches to teaching and to assessment of learning. Library staff may use such software for developing materials for library education programs and user orientations.

Analytical Software

Spreadsheets, statistical packages (such as SAS or SPSS), and database management software may also be useful in the library context for students undertaking research projects or working on papers. Faculty needing such software are more likely to have resources available within their own offices or labs.

Graphics Software

Software that creates graphs, charts, and other illustrative materials, including those that produce slides or overhead transparencies will be greatly appreciated by faculty or staff who teach or make presentations, if these services are not readily available through a biocommunications or publications department. Presentation software that incorporates text, visual, and even audio material offers an easy method for library users and staff to present information for lectures, seminars, or reports.

Even if a library determines that any or all of these types of resources are justified and fit the library's purpose, the question remains about how intensely to acquire them. Typically only one word processing program (or two, if the library has both PCs and Macintosh computers) will be offered, only one graphics program, etc. Decisions may depend on whether the institution uses a standard set of software, has acquired site licenses, offers instruction, and other similar factors. If the library provides classes or demonstrations on a variety of file management software, then it may wish to make each program taught also available for public use.

Sources of Information

Reviews or descriptions of new software programs in the health sciences may be found in *JAMA*, *MD Computing* [10], *Bulletin of the Medical Library Association* and a growing number of publications geared toward information professionals. A summary of medical CD-ROM products reviewed by Hogan in *JAMA* was published in 1993 [11]. *Information Today* includes a section "CD-ROM Today" which contains product information [12]. Other sources are *CD-ROM Professional* and *CD-ROM Librarian* [13-14]. *Library Journal* publishes a regular CD-ROM review column, which sometimes includes health resources, primarily for the public.

The "Library for Internists," published every three years in *Annals of Internal Medicine*, lists a small number of databases and CD-ROM products [15]. In the 1994 edition, most of these entries referred to various forms of MEDLINE, but one would expect the software selections to grow in the future.

To identify programs in the health sciences, selectors might consult the *Software for Health Sciences Education: A Resource Catalog* [16]. Each year *MD-Computing* devotes an issue to its "Annual Medical Hardware and Software Buyers' Guide." Listed by MeSH term, entries consist of vendor-supplied descriptions, including system features and technical information. NLM has published a listing of items in its collection [17]. Two nursing sources include the *AJN Multimedia Catalog* and the *Directory of Educational Software for Nursing* [18-19].

The Lister Hill National Center for Biomedical Communications sponsors an online computer conference network, E.T. Net, that seeks to link users with developers of interactive technology in health science education and encourages participants to share reviews and comments on software. A separate conference, NUCARE (NUrsing CAre REsearch), promotes similar communication for the nursing profession. Numerous interest groups and discussion lists may be identified on the Internet where information about electronic products are shared [20].

More general compilations may be found in *CD-ROMs in Print*, the *CD-ROM Catalog*, and the online directories, *CD-ROM Databases* and *SOFT; Buyer's Guide to Micro Software* [21-24]. A list of health sciences CD-ROM products has been extracted from *CD-ROMS in Print* [25]. This list groups similar resources together, including full text journals, books, and data-bases, subdivided by specialty. Vendors also produce catalogs periodically that list new products of interest to health sciences libraries [26-28].

Information about new software developed for health professional education is described in the annual abstract book that accompanies the Research in Medical Education (RIME) exhibits at the annual meeting of the Association of American Medical Colleges. The voluminous proceedings of the annual *Symposium on Computer Applications in Medical Care* (SCAMC) also describe many new applications. Viewing the proceedings is, of course, a poor substitute for seeing demonstrations and hearing discussions at the meetings themselves.

The Health Sciences Consortium, a consortium of institutions that promotes development of instructional materials in health sciences education, issues catalogs on computer-based education programs, as well as more general medical and allied health catalogs that include computer-based programs [29]. Their catalogs include descriptive information, hardware requirements, and cost. In addition to the catalogs, the Health Sciences Consortium issues a quarterly newsletter and distributes announcements and fliers about individual computer-based education programs.

Selection Process

Most libraries acquiring such software will want to be assured that the product has been assessed positively by subject specialists. In addition to seeking published reviews, recommendations from local users should be obtained; this input may in fact be more crucial to the decision than the external review. It is often possible to get a demonstration version of the software to examine and evaluate. However, unlike review copies of videos or films, demonstration copies of software are often extremely limited and cannot be considered working copies of the software. A more reliable evaluation may be obtained by visiting a site where the software is currently in use.

Because electronic resources may have implications for equipment, library and institutional networks, mainframe resources, system staff requirements, and consortial arrangements, the selection process should include consultation far beyond the decision of a selector, selection committee, or department. If decisions regarding electronic resources are made fairly frequently, the review process should be formalized. A committee, including representatives with knowledge of the system requirements, may be used. If a committee already makes decisions on journals or other materials, the same committee could be expanded when reviewing electronic resources.

Prior review and consultation with the appropriate systems staff, within the library or at a broader level depending on the application and institutional environment, will lay the groundwork for final decision making. Because additional costs for hardware upgrades or support software may be involved, decisions should not be made precipitously without adequate information.

A checklist of criteria to be used in assessing an electronic resource will assure that all the important factors are considered. The published literature should always be checked to determine what experiences others may have reported with a product or application. When there are multiple products that appear to offer roughly the same content, the decision-making process may be more time consuming as a careful comparison of alternatives must be made.

Costs and Budgeting

Computer-based resources have complicated many of the collection decisions in health sciences libraries. Although some advocate "mainstreaming" electronic resources into the collection budget, this approach may take different forms [30]. Which costs should be considered collection costs? Support software costs such as operating systems, menus, use-monitoring software? Hardware costs? Staff support costs to install and maintain?

Both initial and ongoing costs must be considered. In addition to the cost of the software itself, what is the cost of upgrading existing equipment or acquiring new hardware or associated software needed to use the product? Is an annual software maintenance fee required? What are the requirements to acquire new versions as they are released?

When purchasing resources that will be accessed through a network, additional costs must be determined. The producer may offer a network version, or may price the product on the basis of the number of simultaneous users permitted. The amount of use should be estimated in order to determine how many simultaneous users to allow for and to judge whether a network version will be cost-effective.

In order to control costs and encourage a systematic approach to selection, it may be helpful to designate a portion of the collection budget specifically to acquire locally installed electronic resources, even though these resources themselves may fit other budget categories, such as journals or reference materials. As electronic resources become more commonplace, they may be integrated into other collection categories, such as journals, monographs, or subject allocations.

Costs for locally mounted databases such as MEDLINE may also be included within the collection budget. The full costs may encompass not only acquiring or leasing the databases, but storage space and other computer costs. Even if these are not included within the collection budget, they need to be considered when determining the overall cost of providing access to the resource.

Funding Sources

Although basic information resources in electronic formats will be incorporated into the library's collection budget, other sources of funds should not be neglected — especially when they permit experimentation or allow the library to introduce its users to new resources.

Cooperative Endeavors

A number of libraries or institutions may join together to purchase or lease databases that are then made available to their respective users through a common network. Libraries that participate in an integrated library system on a single campus, or share a system within a multicampus system or consortium, have a good opportunity to add databases to the shared system, often with the advantages of linking the bibliographic databases to local library holdings and presenting the user with a single interface.

Cost Sharing

When acquiring subject specific software for which the expected user population is concentrated in a single department or school, shared funding may be considered. A department might support the purchase or if the interest is broader, the cost could be divided among departments. In funding a major resource such as MEDLINE or *Science Citation Index*, a formula could be developed to apportion costs among the various institutional units.

User Charges

Another cost-sharing device is to charge each user for consulting or retrieving information from a resource. The literature is replete with debate over whether to, when to, and how to charge individuals or groups of users. Options include per-use charges, flat rates, block purchases, and other formulas. When weighing alternatives, the institutional environment, the ability and inclination of users to pay for resources, and potential barrier to information charges might impose, will drive the decision.

Staffing and Service

What will be the staff costs to install and maintain the software? How often are updates or new versions expected, and what is the anticipated cost? How much staff time will be anticipated to provide user assistance? Can the library provide that assistance? If not, how high will be the level of user frustration?

Chiang has suggested four potential levels of service [31]:

- Referral: telling requesters where they can find a resource.

- Reference: telling someone about a resource; providing a description or recommendation.

- Consultation: showing someone how to use a resource; providing assistance.

- Instruction: teaching formal classes in use of a resource.

Before making a decision to acquire an electronic resource, the library must agree on what level of support staff should give and whether they can in fact provide it. Does the library have staff who are expert enough to provide consultation? On all applications, or only some? A mix, depending on the resource, is quite possible. For instance, the library staff may teach courses on use of file management software, provide expert assistance with an electronic textbook, give a description and basic introduction to clinical diagnostic software, and refer a requester to another department for a statistical package. The level of support should be determined prior to purchase, following a conscious policy.

Updates, Retention, and Preservation

New Versions

In the same way that print publications are updated with new editions, computer software is updated with new versions. Should the library acquire every new version, especially if updates are not included in the pricing? While the decision is not as simple as choosing to purchase a new edition of a textbook, some of the questions may be the same, such as the extent to which the field has changed, making the content significantly out of date. Additional factors also need to be considered: has the user interface changed? If so, do the changes improve the effectiveness of the product or make it easier to use? Have the memory requirements increased? Will the microcomputers or server on which the software is installed still be adequate? Whatever the answers to these questions, decisions not to acquire updates or revisions should be clearly articulated to library staff and users.

Retention

As with printed publications new versions of electronic resources may supersede earlier editions. Unless the previous version offers content that is still useful and is not contained in the current release, earlier versions of electronic resources will not ordinarily be kept.

The reasons for discarding earlier versions have to do both with technology and with type of use. In common with audiovisual programs, computer-based programs are often created specifically for student use, rather than as more traditional information sources. As learning tools, they should be as up-to-date as possible. Additionally, if the software has seen significant changes in the user interface, it will be confusing to users to have versions that differ noticeably, especially if earlier versions have fewer features. It is also possible that if the library has updated its technology to accommodate new software requirements, older versions may become incompatible with existing equipment. As electronic information resources become more standard and encompass a broader range of uses, research libraries may give more thought to retaining representative versions of selected products.

Preservation

Electronic media have an unknown life-span. Content that has lasting value and that is not available in a more permanent medium may be lost to the future. On the other hand, electronic resources may also provide access to the content or reproduction of older works that might otherwise be unavailable. For many health sciences libraries, with an emphasis on current information and primarily supporting teaching or patient care, archival quality is not an overriding concern. For major research collections, the question of what should be preserved will become more acute as more resources are produced only in electronic form and hardware, software, and operating systems become obsolete at accelerating rates.

Local Productions

Software produced by the local institution will often be made available through the library or associated learning center, especially if used in conjunction with the curriculum. If the library has archival responsibilities or collects books within scope by local authors, it should also consider acquiring significant computer-based products developed within the institution.

Review and Evaluation

Electronic resources should be evaluated on a regular basis. Ongoing commitments need to be reviewed. The library must assess how much and by whom the programs are being used and whether they are serving their intended purpose. Newer products should be reviewed to determine whether the current resource is still the best choice among available resources. Single purchase software should be assessed to assure that it is being used and still provides accurate and current information. If more recent versions are available, they should be evaluated. If a more current version is acquired, the library will need to decide whether to keep previous versions. Except for situations where older information has some value from a historical or research perspective, outdated sources are not likely to prove useful. Collections, electronic as well as print, require regular attention; each library should have a collection assessment plan in place.

Remote Resources: the Global Context

The world of text, image, data, and multimedia information, as well as individual collaborative communications accessible through the Internet, has exploded. This world is changing daily and any textbook discussion will be sadly out of date by the time it reaches the reader. Interfaces and browsers in use today (Gopher, WorldWide Web, Mosaic, NetScape) may be gone tomorrow. The challenge to libraries in general, and collection development in particular, is to find the proper perspective for these far-flung resources, when access can be confusing, erratic, and disorganized as well as fun and full of exciting discoveries.

One method of harnessing remote resources to meet needs of the local institution is to view them as both an extension of the library's collections and as an integral part of it, applying similar criteria for selecting and providing easy access. Riley and Shipman have described a process of "resource discovery," resource evaluation, and menu design [32]. In the resource discovery phase, potential resources are identified through list-servs, newsgroups, and Internet resource guides. Following discovery, resources are evaluated using criteria similar to those for electronic re-sources: perceived quality; relevance to local activity and interest; "fit" with local/available relationship to other library resources; and evidence of ongoing maintenance. Selected resources, which have been screened and recommended are added to the institution's local menu of resources, facili-tating easy access by users.

Not only do the individual information resources accessible through the Internet continually appear and disappear, but so do the network sites that point users to them, through such programs as Gopher or World Wide Web (WWW). Because of the transient nature of these resources, only two electronic directories are mentioned here. Both are interdisciplinary direc-tories listing a wide variety of Internet resources: *Clearinghouse for Subject Oriented Internet Resources Guide* (Ann Arbor: University of Michigan, http//WWW.lib.umich.edu/chrome.html) and *Yahoo* (http://WWW.Ya-hoo.com/Health). A subject directory has also been published in paper form [33].

Identification, evaluation, and ongoing monitoring of remote resources can be incorporated into collection development responsibilities. Selection guidelines developed for local collections can be adapted to address the unique aspects of Internet or other remote resources [34-35]. By selecting particular resources and guiding users to them through local information systems, the library plays an important role in making the vast world of accessible resources more responsive to institutional priorities and individ-ual user needs.

References

1. Bosch S, Promis P, Sugnet C. Guide to selecting and acquiring CD-ROMs, software, and other electronic publications. Chicago: American Library Association, 1994. (Acquisitions guidelines no. 9).

2. Morse DH, Richards DT. Collection development policies for health sciences libraries. Chicago: Medical Library Association, 1992. (MLA DocKit no. 3).

3. Taylor CR. Great expectations: the reading habits of year II medical students. New Engl J Med 1992 May 21; 326(21):1436-40.

4. Demas S. Collection development for the electronic library: a conceptual and organizational model. Libr Hi Tech 1994; 12(3):71-80.

5. Berner ES et al. Performance of four computer-based diagnostic systems. New Engl J Med 1994 Jun 23; 330(25):1792 - 1826.

6. Elliot R, ed. MEDLINE on CD-ROM; National Library of Medicine evaluation forum. Medford, NJ: Learned Information, 1989.

7. Boss RW. Accessing electronic publications in complex LAN environments. Libr Technol Rep 1992 May-Jun;28(3):311-20.

8. Hannigan GG, Brown JF. Managing public access microcomputers in health sciences libraries. Chicago: Medical Library Association, 1990.

9. Cramer MD. Licensing agreements: think before you act. Coll Res Libr News 1994 Sep; 55(8): 496-7.

10. MD Computing. Bimonthly. New York: Springer Verlag.

11. Hogan R. Medical CD-ROMs. JAMA 1993 Oct 6; 270(13): 1613.

12. Information Today. Monthly. Medford, NJ: Learned Information.

13. CD-ROM Professional. Bimonthly. Weston, CT: Pemberton Press.

14. CD-ROM Librarian. Bimonthly. Westport, CT: Meckler.

15. Mazza JJ. A library for internists VIII. Recommendations from the American College of Physicians. Ann Intern Med 1994 Apr 15;120(8):699-720.

16. Software for Health Sciences Education: a resource catalog. 6th ed. Ann Arbor, MI: Learning Resources Center, Office of Medical Education, University of Michigan Medical Center, 1995.

17. NLM Catalog of Publications, Audiovisuals, and Software. Bethesda, MD: National Library of Medicine. 1995.

18. AJN Multimedia Catalog. New York: American Journal of Nursing Company, 1994.

19. Bolwell C. Directory of Educational Software for Nursing. 5th ed. New York: National League for Nursing, 1993. (Publ. no. 41-2553).

20. King LA, Kovacs D. Directory of electronic journals, newsletters and academic discussion lists. 4th ed. Washington, D.C.: Association of Research Libraries, 1994.

21. CD-ROMs in Print; an international guide to CD-ROM, CD-I, 3DO, MMCD, CD32, multimedia and electronic book products. Annual. Westport, CT: Meckler Media.

22. CD-ROM Catalog. Annual. Los Angeles, CA: Updata Publications (http:www.updata.com).

23. CD-ROM Databases. Monthly. Boston: Worldwide Videotex.

24. SOFT; Buyer's Guide to Micro Software. (Distributed through BRS, Dialog).

25. Chiang D. CD-ROMs in health sciences libraries. Med Ref Serv. Quart. 1993 Summer; 12(2): 67-81.

26. CD-ROM Handbook. Birmingham, AL: Ebsco Subscription Services.

27. Faxon guide to CD-ROM. Boston: The Faxon Company.

28. Multimedia catalog. Dallas: J.A. Majors.

29. Computer-based Education Catalog. Chapel Hill, NC: Health Sciences Consortium, 1995.

30. Demas S. Software and collection development. Pt. I Mainstreaming software. Tech Serv Quart 1990; 7(3): 13-16.

31. Chiang K. Software and collection development. Pt. II Services and staff skills. Tech Serv Q 1990; 7(3): 17-20.

32. Riley RA, Shipman BL. Building and maintaining a library gopher: traditional skills applied to emerging resources. Bull Med Libr Assoc 1995 Apr; 83(2): 221-7.

33. Internet resources: a subject guide. Chicago: Association of College and Resource Libraries, 1995.

34. Demas S, McDonald P, Lawrence G. The Internet and collection development: mainstreaming selection of Internet resources. Libr Res Tech Serv 1995 Jul; 39(3): 275-90.

35. Cassel R. Selection criteria for Internet resources. Coll Res Libr News 1995 Feb; 56(2): 92-3.

7

Selection in Special Settings

"There are times when I think the ideal library is composed solely of reference books. They are like understanding friends, always ready to change the subject when you have had enough of this or that."

J. Donald Adams, 1956

Health sciences libraries exist to serve a range of user interests. Consequently, the collections and emphases in those collections can and will vary significantly from library to library. There is great similarity among collections that support an academic curriculum in the health sciences or in libraries where the focus of the collection is research in a particular field such as pharmaceuticals. One expects the collections to contain a high percentage of the same materials. While most libraries will hold a common core collection of book and journal titles that focus on the health sciences generally, those libraries will also have reference collections to support information services. The selection process for reference materials requires the consideration of additional criteria before making a decision. Collections that support research in historical health sciences topics or that provide assistance and information to health care consumers are assembled with different criteria in mind.

In each of these special settings, there are special concerns in the collection development process, principally in selection of materials, which are different from collection development for general book and journal collections. The generic criteria described in Chapter 4, Polices and Criteria, and elaborated on in Chapters 5, Selection: Journals and Books, and Chapter 6, Selection: Electronic Resources, will apply to selection in special settings, though the emphasis and applicability may vary. Further, there are some specialized selection sources which will be of interest. The following sections consider briefly some of the differences in collection development for reference collections, audiovisual collections, consumer health collections, and rare book and history of medicine collections. As has been stated elsewhere in this volume, the aim is not to be comprehensive but rather to introduce the topic. The references at the end of this chapter cover in greater depth the specific concerns of collection development in these settings. Finally, Appendix B includes examples of collection development policy statements for these special settings. Additional examples may be found in the MLA DocKit [1].

Reference Collections

Although reference service continues as an expected role for health sciences libraries, the traditional reference desk, staffed long hours by reference librarians, with nearby collections of printed indexes, directories, and other reference works becomes less and less the norm. As budgets shrink, priorities change, and libraries evaluate their use of staff, more front-line help may be given by library assistants or other support staff, while librarians may be on call or available by appointment only. Nonetheless, questions continue to be asked, the library staff continue to provide answers, and the concept of a need for a reference collection continues.

The policy for the reference collection should relate to the policy for the general collection. However, the reference collection is not necessarily a microcosm of the general collection and should not be regarded as a distillation of it. For this reason, establishing a policy and selection criteria for the reference collection is particularly important. Examples of reference collection policies are found in Appendix B.

Readers are referred to the text by Roper and Boorkman for a more detailed discussion of reference collections and review of specific works [2]. Only general principles are outlined here.

Purpose

The main purpose of a reference collection is efficiency. By separating selected materials into a distinct location, convenient for library staff, and restricting its use to on-site consultation, users' questions can be answered more speedily and successfully than if the reference materials were integrated into the rest of the collection. On the other hand, in a library with a large well-stocked reference section, there is danger that staff will restrict their search for answers to the materials at hand. The entire collection, as well as sources beyond the bounds of the library, constitute the true reference collection. In most libraries, heavy use by staff for answering user queries and the need for constant availability should dictate which materials are chosen for a reference collection, rather than the type of material.

Reference collections have numerous functions. Before developing a specific policy, the library staff making selection decisions should determine the degree to which these functions are important in their particular setting. Reference works are commonly used to locate the following:

- *Directory Information:* Brief factual information about people, institutions, organizations, programs.

- *Data:* Compilations of such information as statistical data, biological facts, chemical composition, drug descriptions.

- *Definitions:* Collections of medical terminology, foreign languages, specialized nomenclature.

- *Descriptions:* Short or encyclopedic summaries of diseases, procedures, biological processes, historical events.

- *Bibliographic Information:* References or abstracts by subject, author, citation, historical period, or source.

Selection Criteria

Criteria for selecting reference works may differ considerably from those criteria for the collection in general. The subject scope will be broader, encompassing directories, reference texts, and even indexes for subjects that may be peripheral to the main collection. For example, a handbook of chemistry may be acquired for the reference collection even if chemistry journals are considered out of scope. A directory of research grants, a manual of government agencies, a German dictionary, an encyclopedia of science—all may be highly useful for reference purposes, but peripheral to the general collection. On the other hand, while the scope may be very broad, the types of materials collected are quite specific and highly selective, and the reference collection should parallel the general collection in areas of emphasis and subject depth.

The factors that influence selection of materials for a reference collection are similar to those for the general collection, but are evaluated more intensely because these are the sources of first resort for answering users' questions. If the search goes no further, the first answer should be the correct or best one.

Authority

How accurate is the information likely to be? For statistics or other data, what is their source? Does the compilation constitute an official publication? Are directories issued by authoritative bodies? Does the textbook represent the accepted standard for current knowledge and practice? Does the drug information come from pharmaceutical companies or regulatory bodies? Are publishers, editors, authors reputable?

Currency

Where was the work compiled, written, or published? To be useful, a reference collection must be current. Libraries with very limited budgets that have access to other collections, such as a general university or nearby public library, may choose not to purchase every edition of some general reference works. For works in which the content does not change rapidly, such as organization directories or language dictionaries, it may not be critical to have every new edition. A cooperative arrangement may be worked out with another library usually on the same campus in the same institution or within a consortium to receive the previous edition when another library purchases a new one. A pair of libraries may also decide that they will reduce costs by each ordering alternate editions, staggering purchases so the latest edition is always available in one of the two libraries.

For medical information that becomes dated, not having the latest version can be a hazard. Reference works with drug information, for example, should be as current as possible. Directories of individuals or compilations of medical statistical data should also be kept current.

Comprehensiveness

How thoroughly does the bibliography or index cover the literature? How selective is the directory? How inclusive is the dictionary or handbook? Does the content depend on voluntary contributions?

Consultability

How easily can the publication or database be consulted? Is the organization logical and the index comprehensive?

Usefulness

How often is the resource likely to be used? How essential is it to have immediately available? How critical is the information it contains?

Textbook Collections

The physical organization of the library, the makeup of its primary user population, the nature and placement of its reserve collection, and whether it has a noncirculating collection of standard textbooks will guide the decision whether to include medical texts in the reference collection. Textbooks are used as sources for short authoritative answers to reference questions. They also frequently contain basic historical information for the specialty or topic. A representative collection of textbooks in the reference collection may provide convenient access to students who need information for assignments or patient care questions.

Electronic Resources

Library reference collections include electronic as well as print sources. A more detailed discussion will be found in the chapter on "Microcomputers and Reference Service" by Brown and Hannigan in Volume 1 of this series, *Reference and Information Services in Health Sciences Libraries* [3]. With the growth of online databases and electronic storage devices, such as optical disc, CD-ROM, and computer diskettes, reference sources are now accessible through a wide variety of media. Print indexes may have disappeared, online directories may be more up to date, and hypertext programs may allow more precise searching. In some cases, paper copies are retained only because the publisher's pricing policies favor acquiring both paper and electronic formats. Multiple access points, Boolean logic, keyword searching, and hypertext capabilities give clear advantage to electronic formats for locating bibliographic information. For most queries they are more efficient and more effective. Imagine choosing to consult the recent monthly issues of *Index Medicus* rather than searching MEDLINE!

Although electronic formats often offer search and display features not possible in print publications, the hardware and software requirements can pose certain disadvantages. *Current Contents* on disk, the *Physicians Desk Reference* (PDR) on stand alone CD-ROM, *Micromedex* on the hospital's local area network, the *NIH Guide* on the campus network, and GenBank through the Internet illustrate the array of media that must be navigated by reference staff. Multiple equipment and software requirements, sign-on protocols, and search commands combine to create strains on library budgets as well as staff time for installation, maintenance, updating, and training. Faulty equipment, as well as system and power failures, cut off access. Without high-grade multitasking computers and easy-to-use menus for various resources, access can take more time and effort for a quick look-up question than going to a printed directory or compendium.

Criteria for selecting electronic resources are discussed more generally in Chapter 6. Highlighted here are factors that should be weighed in evaluating electronic reference sources.

1. Does the electronic format offer features that clearly improve the product's usefulness?
2. How easy is it to use? Does it require training or is searching intuitive?
3. How frequently is it updated? How easy are updates to install? Does the library have staff to handle updates promptly?
4. Does the library have the equipment required by the resource? Will it require additional memory, network access, a different program platform or other software for quick response time and effective display?
5. Will the resource have to be accessible on dedicated equipment or does it require rebooting or multiple steps to move from another application on the same machine before access to the resource is possible?
6. How does the cost compare with the comparable print publication or with other similar electronic resources?
7. Will the resource be available for use by the public as well as by reference staff? Will it be convenient? Will users require assistance? Will staff be available to provide it?
8. Does the publisher impose restrictive license agreements that conflict with library policies or create barriers to reasonable access?

Ephemeral Material

Collections of pamphlets, information sheets, brochures, and even reprints or bibliographies are maintained by some libraries as adjuncts to reference collections. If such a collection is maintained, the library should have a clear policy on what types of material it collects and why. Pamphlet collections can become depositories for little used "stuff" that was determined not to be of sufficiently lasting value for the permanent collection, but that "someone might want." Such collections can also consume staff time, especially if content records are created and maintained. Collections of brochure-type information may be useful if the library serves the general public or patients. A clippings file of current news items related to medicine and health generally, or about the local scene and institution, might have value in certain settings. Regardless of the purpose, the library should have a policy that includes selection criteria and guidelines for weeding and retention. The policy should then be followed.

Duplication

Unless the reference collection includes a core collection of medical textbooks and the library either maintains a separate reserve collection or needs circulating copies of textbooks, most materials in the reference collection will be the library's only copy. The very nature of most reference material implies it is used for "reference," that is, consultation, and additional copies in the general collection are unlikely to be needed.

Resource Sharing

Reference works, especially large sets, can be very costly. When the need to consult such sources is infrequent, the library may consider cooperative approaches to access—sharing the cost with other libraries in the same institution to provide a single copy on campus; acquiring one set for consortium use; or relying on the regional medical library or a designated resource library within the region to provide backup reference assistance.

Retention and Weeding

Because its purpose is to meet demands for current primarily factual information, a reference collection requires frequent review and weeding. Only the most recent edition of most directories, dictionaries, and other periodically updated works will be kept in the reference collection. Library records, such as the public catalog, should reflect this policy and indicate the location of earlier editions kept by the library. If such publications are maintained on a standing order with the publisher or a vendor to automatically receive new editions, check-in records should alert library staff with instructions to replace the current edition.

Should a library keep earlier editions of reference materials? The answer to this question depends on the purpose and role of the library and its relationship to other local collections. A hospital library designed to serve the present needs of physicians, hospital staff, and students for information related to patient care will find little reason to retain out-of-date reference materials. On the other hand, a large academic health sciences library centered in a heavily research-oriented institution may serve as a site for historical information, which, although rarely needed, is invaluable to a researcher. One who is tracing the history of an individual or examining the evolution of medical terminology or changes in prescription data over time may well need to consult older editions.

Even in libraries with a role in preserving historical information, retention should not be indiscriminate. Outdated reference works in fields other than the health sciences should rarely be kept, especially if the institution has a general research library. With rare exceptions there is no need to retain every edition of a frequently updated work. A representative collection, for example, an edition every five years, will serve most purposes.

The decision to weed a publication from the reference collection does not mean that the work should not be kept by the library or that it no longer has reference value. A particular work may no longer be consulted frequently and though it contains unique information, it may be dated or no longer relevant to current needs. Shifting lesser used items to the regular collection concentrates the reference collection and makes it easier to use for quick responses to information queries.

Responsibility for Selection

In libraries with a separate reference or information services staff, selection of materials for the reference collection normally falls to someone in that unit. Those who are directly involved in providing reference assistance are generally best qualified to determine the resources needed.

Reference staff should also make recommendations or decisions regarding whether older editions should be kept by the library. There should be a process and schedule of periodically reviewing the collection and removing publications that do not meet criteria for frequent consultation or need for constant availability. (For additional information on reference collections, refer to Volume 1 in this series, *Reference and Information Services in Health Sciences Libraries.*)

Audiovisual Collections

Audiovisual materials comprise an important segment of many health sciences libraries. Their importance in medicine has long been recognized, especially as alternatives to prose descriptions, and for their use in health professional education. These collections have requirements (such as space, equipment, and funding) that make them different from collections of other materials. A very useful resource written to provide guidance for reference materials in this area, but which covers many other aspects of AV librarianship in a health sciences setting, is Futrelle and Curtis' chapter in Roper and Boorkman [4].

Audiovisuals have unique features which secure their place in library collections, in particular the ability of individual formats to convey difficult or complex concepts more effectively and efficiently than their print counterparts. Examples include the auscultation and other sounds of physiological phenomena on an audiotape, the merger of sound and graphics to create an operating room environment on a videotape, and the three-dimensional aspects of models in conveying anatomical principles. There may also be staffing implications for audiovisual collections and special requirements for proper storage. Further, there is a heightened focus on current materials so "It is important to use frequently updated and current reference sources . . ."[5].

Especially important to some collections are works which document medical innovations, procedures, attitudes, social issues or policies concerning or affecting health care. Other important audiovisual materials are those which record significant events in the life and work of individuals or institutions important in the health sciences. Contemporary examples of authoritative items designed to demonstrate surgical procedures may be found in health sciences library collections. Local productions, including those made by hospital audiovisual services, are common items in hospital libraries, as are downloaded broadcasts from Hospital Satellite Network (HSN) and other telecommunication networks. Even though selected items are important in some collections, many have a short life span in terms of interest and usefulness.

An audiovisual component in a health sciences library may operate under different or the same guidelines as those which prevail for the parent library. "Nonprint collections are generally characterized as 'working collections'"[6] and are typically assembled to support some kind of educational mission. Whichever is the case, the service and the collection should be responsive to the needs of the users, whether that is medical education, patient education, clinical support, or continuing medical education.

A significant difference in collection development for audiovisuals is the selection process itself, which is usually more user-driven than that for other formats. That is, the faculty member or instructor who will use or assign the audiovisual item frequently is an active participant in the selection process. Indeed, many libraries do not select materials for an audiovisual collection without the express involvement of the person who will incorporate the material into an educational session. Patient education coordinators may participate in the identification and review of audiovisual titles, as may personnel specialists, hospital administrators, and other types of users.

The second aspect of the selection process, which is a departure from common practice, is the preview. Many audiovisual producers permit or rent an individual title to an institution so that the title can be previewed to determine if it is sufficiently relevant to warrant a purchase. Typically, the library's audiovisual department can arrange a preview, during which the requesting user is expected to make detailed analyses of the title before a selection decision is made.

It is also important for the library to incorporate into its collection development policy for audiovisuals a statement reflecting its consortial arrangements. Such arrangements can expand the number of items which may be available to the user group and may stimulate cooperative collection development.

Purpose

As noted earlier, an audiovisual collection in a health sciences library, whether in an academic setting or in a hospital, typically supports some type of educational program. Audiovisuals are used in the education of health professionals at the undergraduate and graduate level and are also important components of continuing medical education programs in hospitals and medical centers. Audiovisual formats facilitate self-study and can be meaningful parts of in-service training programs.

As with books and other resources, audiovisual materials may also be collected to meet a patient education need, either for teaching self-care to a patient or to instruct a patient's family about a particular diagnosis or disease. Audiovisuals can be very useful as well in assisting patients to become aware of the options for treatment for a disease.

Selection Criteria

As with other material selection, the process should be a weighing of factors, one against or with another, to reach a decision. In addition to the general criteria for selection discussed in Chapter 4, the following additional criteria may be considered in selecting audiovisuals. These criteria may be augmented by local practice.

Audience

Is the audience for which the audiovisual is produced part of the library's user group? Audiovisuals are typically produced for a professional audience, for academics, or for the general public, including patients and patient families. This factor is described in brochures and most other selection sources. The library's interest in these audiences should be carefully documented in the collection development policy and taken into account in the selection process.

Equipment Availability

Does the library already own the proper equipment so that users can view or listen to the program? If the answer is negative, what is the likelihood that additional titles in the particular format will be acquired in the future? Are users likely to have access to compatible equipment at home or in their departments? Can the item be used on patient or other broadcast networks? Many libraries began to purchase VHS videotapes when that format became a popular standard for home use.

Appropriateness of Format

Is the format in which the material is presented the most useful one to convey the information? For example, presentation of cytology stains may be more effective in a slide format than in a videotape format because the former will permit the student to study the individual slide at an individual pace. Further, some information is enhanced in an audiovisual format and may be preferred to a print presentation. If motion is integral to the information being conveyed, a still image is not the best way to present the information. The actual sounds of the heart and lung are easier to grasp through an audiotape than by reading a printed description.

Origin of Format

Does the audiovisual conform to national standards? Audiovisuals produced outside the United States sometimes do not conform to U.S. equipment standards. Videotapes are a prime example of this. Slides as well may be of different sizes than those which are produced in this country.

Rental or Permanent Acquisition

Can the need for the particular item be satisfied through a one-time rental? Is there sufficient recurring demand to warrant a purchase?

Restrictions on Use

Are there special guidelines which must be followed regarding the use of the title, such as a prohibition on group showings? If it is difficult to monitor and enforce such restrictions, it may not be advisable to purchase the item.

Cost

Is the item worth the investment? Audiovisuals are often designed for group use but can be used by individuals as well. As such, the typically high expenditure may be more easily justified because more individuals will use the item.

Retention and Weeding

Most audiovisuals have a shorter shelf life than print materials. For this reason, they are typically not retained as permanent parts of a collection. Audiovisual collections should be subjected to regular review to identify appropriate items for removal.

Like the selection process, the weeding process should be governed by specialized criteria. Each of the above criteria can be a factor in the deselection decision and should be considered. Additional criteria include the following.

Obsolescence of Format

Are materials still being produced in the format? The filmstrip, for example, is rarely used these days and the slide-tape presentation is quickly being replaced by videotape.

Outdated Content

Is the operation or laboratory technique that is the subject of the audiovisual still being used? Has the educational emphasis of the user group for which the item was initially selected changed? Have other items in the collection superseded this item or rendered it redundant?

Presentation Style

Are the settings or the clothing worn by the actors of another era? Though the message may still be valid, outmoded production values may interfere with the educational message of an instructional program.

Selection Sources

A large proportion of audiovisuals in medicine have been produced by organizations, educational institutions and the like: a significant difference between audiovisuals and printed resources. "Information about available audiovisual . . . software appears first in the brochures and catalogs of the producers and distributors of health sciences media"[7]. This presents some specific selection concerns because information about medical audiovisuals is not as systematic as their print counterparts. There are approximately seventy-five major print publishers in the health sciences and more than 1,000 media producers.

There is no single guide for medical audiovisuals, though there are several tools which can be useful to identify titles for consideration. Futrelle and Curtis review and describe in detail the primary audiovisual reference sources[8]. Primary among these are AVLINE, NLM's online database of audiovisuals in the health sciences. This source contains bibliographic information for more than 55,000 audiovisuals and frequently provides loan and price data [9]. Among the most valuable aspects of this tool are its abstracts.

The primary print counterpart to AVLINE was the *NLM Audiovisuals Catalog* [10] which can still be useful for retrospective selection and for comparative selection because of its subject index, which brings items in a specific subject together. The audiovisual serials index is another important feature. This publication ceased in 1993 but access to AVLINE continues through a variety of electronic means.

A-V Online [11] offers access to information about several thousand educational audiovisuals, including health sciences titles. This database is available in several formats and can be searched through major database services. Many other databases include information about health sciences audiovisuals and can be used as selection sources.

Other important general audiovisual print directories which may be helpful for selection are the *Educational Film & Video Locator* [12] which has "established itself as an indispensable reference tool for identifying audiovisual materials to rent" [13], and the *Video Source Book* [14], the most recent edition of which contains information about 126,000 audiovisual programs. The National Information Center for Educational Media (NICEM) provides information for a series of guides, *Film & Video Finder* [15], *Audiocassette & Compact Disc Finder* [16], and *Filmstrip & Slide Set Finder* [17], each of which contains health sciences titles. The principal sources for producer addresses and other information about the audiovisual market-place are *AV Market Place* [18], and the *Index to AV Producers & Distributors* [19], now in its 9th edition.

Reviews constitute another important source for information about new audiovisual titles in the biomedical sciences. The two most significant titles which publish reviews are *Media Profiles: the Health Sciences Edition* [20] and *Health Media Review Index* [21]. *Media Profiles: the Health Sciences Edition* combines original reviews prepared by health professionals with extensive content information. *Health Media Review Index*, by contrast, is an index which compiles and abstracts reviews appearing in a wide range of peri-odicals and other sources. Both of these titles can be very useful in the collection development process for audiovisual collections.

A process that uses a variety of sources and that involves the ultimate user intimately in the selection process can result in a very dynamic and well-used audiovisual collection in most health sciences libraries.

Consumer Health Collections

Contemporary health care practice generally seeks to enlist patient involvement and participation in the prevention and management of dis-eases and the maintenance of health. It also seeks to involve families, caregivers, and others not traditionally thought of as health care profession-als in the prevention, intervention, and management of serious conditions. These factors imply certain consideration for the selector in choosing materials that fit the particular setting, philosophy, audience, and use patterns that the library supports.

The demand for consumer health information has risen dramatically in recent years. Wilderness and environmental medicine, mind or body puri-fication, the path to medical discoveries, quackery, health risks of comput-ing, medical technology, herbalism, choosing the best doctor, and the rise of for-profit hospital "chains" have all been the topics of recent new books. So too have more familiar topics, such as wellness, health professional education, national health care reform, and homeopathy. Several medical center-sponsored family health guides, some specialized, others general, have made their debut to share library shelves with standard titles spon-sored by major health associations. There is substantial interest too in disease specific personal narratives, aging, family planning, AIDS, birth techniques, child development, allergies, and the social aspects of health care. The high level of publication of books in nutrition, diet therapy, fitness and exercise, parenting, and child care continues.

Books on all of these subjects may be found in consumer health collections. Audiovisual materials intended to inform health care consumers about specific diseases and conditions, treatment options, medications, and problems of coping with chronic diseases are also included. Materials on basic wellness and nutrition may be collected, as well as a representative selection of material on alternative medical treatments. A few dictionaries, encyclopedias, and directories will generally be included in a consumer health collection. Indexes to consumer health literature will be available in print and computerized formats. *Health Reference Center* [22] a CD-ROM-based consumer health information resource, provides access to an extensive collection of journal articles and pamphlets through both indexing and full text.

In addition to commercially available books, there are many disease specific associations and organizations that have as a principal goal the education of the public about the disease. These groups publish booklets and pamphlets that provide succinct and clearly written explanations of the medical background and treatment for the disease. This type of publication is frequently distributed in single copies free or at little charge. Lists of such organizations can be found in several of the general reference books in a library's reference collection.

The education of the nation's "health conscience" requires authoritative, reliable and comprehensible information and more and more, the health consumer is turning to the library for that information. The heightened involvement of the health consumer in determining the choices associated with health care is predicated on access to comprehensible discussions of frequently complex subjects and issues. Television specials on health issues and specific diseases have created a demand for supplementary readings written for the general public.

Purpose

Consumer health collections exist to serve library users seeking authoritative information, in clearly understood language, about normal anatomy and physiology, diseases, conditions, treatments, and other health care topics. Kernaghan [23] and Rees [24] discuss in detail the place and role of consumer health collections in health sciences libraries. Besides the general public, users of these collections include medical school students seeking materials to help explain health and disease concepts to patients and families. Primary care physicians and nurses, as well as health professional school faculty members, may seek out such materials. Patients, either on referral from a health professional or on their own, seek resources to explain health and disease concepts to families, or to learn more about a diagnosis for themselves. In some hospital settings, the consumer health collection is an integral part of the hospital's public relations effort and is maintained as a magnet for patients. Indeed, in some of these settings, the consumer health collection is not a part of the health sciences library at all.

Health sciences libraries that contain collections of materials aimed at the health care consumer or the patient typically do so as part of a broader institutional educational mission, that is, patient education, or to meet the information needs of the general public. A library may choose not to include works written for this audience, either because of institutional restrictions or because other libraries (such as public libraries) are considered more appropriate locations for this type of information. Libraries that have established collections containing information specifically produced for this audience typically concentrate on works about the functioning of the normal, healthy body, its organs and their functions, the physiological aspects of human development, the maintenance of health, and similar kinds of materials on major diseases.

One very useful guide [25] to establishing a telephone-based consumer health information service in a hospital environment recommends that the following materials be in the collection.

1. Several basic, up-to-date medical texts as well as consumer-oriented medical information sources.
2. A vertical file collection that contains clippings from current periodicals.
3. A computer that permits access to various information databases, maintains the service management files, and contains physician referral lists.

Selection Criteria

The focus in collection development is usually to select authoritative and informative titles as well as a representative number of works to introduce a topic. The general selection criteria, which appear in Chapter 4, are useful for selection of materials for consumer health collections. Further considerations and criteria include the following.

Presentation of Information

Is the writing style appropriate for the information being conveyed and for the health consumer? Is the information easy to find? Does the book include a good index or table of contents? Are the illustrations appropriate? Does it present alternatives that would be useful for making informed decisions about health issues and medical services? Is the information supported by citations and sources?

Audience

Is the audience for which the book is written part of the library's user group? Consumer health materials are typically written for the general public. They may also be written to assist the health professional in conveying information to patients. The library's interest in these audiences should be carefully documented in the collection development policy and taken into account in the selection process.

Pathways to Additional Information

Does the item contain bibliographies, reading lists, referral sources, resource organizations?

Qualifications of the Author and Publisher

Does the author have relevant academic credentials and authoritative institutional affiliations? Is the publisher a reputable one in this field? Has the publisher issued other works designed for consumer health collections?

Currency

How current is the information presented? Are the citations up to date?

Retention and Weeding

Currency of the consumer health collection should be maintained through a regular program of selection, acquisition, and weeding. Because the focus of the collection is current, authoritative material, most materials will have been published within the last five years. Items older than five years should be reviewed periodically to determine their continued usefulness in the collection.

Selection Sources

An important source for titles on consumer health topics is Rees' *Consumer Health Information Source Book* [26], useful because of its voluminous coverage and its critical abstracts. Rees has also prepared a very useful collection of many important U.S. government produced consumer health publications [27]. Selection can also be based on reviews in the professional library literature, such as *Library Journal* and *Choice*, or recommendations from hospital consumer and patient health education providers. Newspapers and popular magazines sometimes carry feature articles about popular medicine titles. *The Reader's Adviser* [28], a multivolume publication designed for public libraries, contains chapters of annotated citations of books on medicine and health and illness and disease. Several booksellers issue periodic catalogs containing lists of books written explicitly for the health care consumer. Bookstores, to accommodate the wealth of publications in this area, frequently have reading alcoves where these materials may be examined. Lastly, physicians often can suggest publications that in their experience have been of help to their patients.

Rare Book and History of Medicine Collections

Rare book and history of medicine collections are not found in all health sciences libraries, but outstanding examples of such collections exist in all types of health sciences libraries. The principal difference between collection development for general health sciences library collections and for rare book collections derives from the nature of the books themselves. Rare books are by definition less common than most of the other books in medical library collections. The level of bibliographic description for rare books is much more extensive, and the condition of many rare books is cause for additional concern at the point of selection.

Because of the generally high value and public relations importance of historical and archival collections, and the highly idiosyncratic nature of these collections, the policies guiding development of them frequently are singled out for special consideration in overall collection development policy statements. Idiosyncrasies in rare book collections may derive from specific donors or donations which shaped the collection, from historical emphases on formats or subjects, or from changing academic interests. Other factors which affect the collection include the age, value, and attention of previous library staff and faculty. Rare book collection development is usually a more scholarly endeavor with typically fewer acquisitions than in other types of collections. Further, the goals of the collection may be quite different and more restricted than those for the overall collection. Overmier has observed that "Medical rare book collections must have extraordinarily long term goals. It may take 20 years to find a specific book" [29].

Funding for rare book collection development departs from funding for other types of collection development. There is a greater reliance on endowed or gift funding as well as a greater dependence on gifts of individual items and collections. A common practice in rare book collections is turning gift duplicates that are not needed or appropriate for the collection into ready cash for the purchase of other books. This is generally done either through trusted dealers who may establish a credit for the library or through outright sale by auction or list prepared by the library.

Overmier has further stated that

> ...the community of medical rare book collections is a small but vigorous one. Medical rare book librarians are moving rapidly toward modern collection development models, particularly with regard to written policies that formalize their traditional practices [30].

Zinn, in her *Handbook* chapter on special collections, observes that "One of the most important activities and perhaps the most time-consuming for a librarian responsible for historical and special collections is the selection and acquisition of appropriate materials" [31]. She suggests that the most important tool in that process is the collection development policy that guides the process. The policy statement should flow from that of the overall library collection, but should include more descriptive information about the holdings of the rare book collection than for the general collection.

Most rare book collection development complements the strengths of a general collection and is based on the type of service that the collection is intended to support. A collection in which active scholarship is being performed will require a different developmental approach than a collection that is principally a reference collection. Zinn's chapter provides a thoughtful analysis of the many issues that must go into the writing of a collection development policy statement for a rare book collection [32].

A distinction is often made between rare book collections and history of medicine collections, under the assumption that the latter are generally comprised of secondary works. These materials may be collected in much the same manner as other books for the medical library collection and are housed in open stacks with the rest of the library's collection. In actual practice, however, most history of medicine collections are a combination of primary and secondary works, both rare and current, housed in close proximity for ease of use.

Rare books are most frequently regarded as primary research materials and housed in rooms with better temperature and humidity controls and security than the general stack collection. A rare book collection may also be a showpiece for the institution and may serve as a magnet for attracting donations from alumni and other interested collectors. Most rare book collections have some type of specialization, though some are still developed along broad subjects paralleling the general medical library.

A significant component of any rare book or history of medicine collection is the reference collection that supports it. This support is necessary to provide quality reference service and to allow the librarian to respond to a broad range of information requests. All health sciences libraries contain a reference collection for historical topics though the books which comprise that collection may not have been assembled with that purpose in mind. Historical information can be found in dictionaries of all types, bibliographies, biographical sources, statistical compilations, books on books, indexing and abstracting services, the introductions to textbooks, and occasional articles in periodicals. This type of collection was characterized as a "ghost" historical reference collection by Kubinec and Richards [33]. They also describe the components of three levels for historical reference collections: basic, intermediate, and research.

Rare book collections may also assume some responsibility for archival materials, especially those publications issued by the primary parent institution. Such materials include catalogs, alumni publications, newsletters, and, sometimes, official documents and policies of the institution. Publications from members of the staff and from other local health-related organizations, such as affiliated hospitals, may be of interest.

Purpose

Rare book and history of medicine collections are generally found in health sciences libraries serving institutions that foster scholarship or education in the history of medicine. The purpose for these collections therefore is to support those activities. Such collections may also be held simply because the institution is old and the library has been in existence for many years. In this case an active collection development program is unusual.

Selection Criteria

Rare book collection development policies contain more historical information about the collection, its strengths and weaknesses, than do general collection development policies. One typically finds descriptions of named collections presented by benefactors. These documents also are more detailed and specific with regard to subjects of interest and scope of collecting.

The generic criteria articulated in Chapter 4 may be applied in the selection of rare books and historical materials. Additional criteria which are considered in that process include the following.

Presence of Other Editions of the Same Work

Are other editions or printings of the book already in the collection? In contrast to a current general health sciences library collection that is usually seeking the most recent edition of a work, multiple editions of older medical books are acquired for rare book collections because these earlier editions have historical value in tracing the origin of medical procedures and discoveries. For rare book collecting, one may also be looking for an earlier edition, such as the first because it is the first, or the second, because typically that is the one in which the greatest number of changes occur, or some other edition with some special feature. Scholarship may require that all editions of a work be acquired for comparison.

Availability of a Facsimile Edition

Is a facsimile of the original edition available? Facsimile editions reproduce the original text and frequently contain historical commentary, a bibliographic history of the work, and a census of holding libraries of the original. Facsimiles can be very useful as reading copies, as copies to be consulted when it is inappropriate or impossible to consult an original, and as a complement to worn or incomplete originals.

Physical Condition

Is the prospective purchase in good physical condition? Because of their age, the paper, binding, and illustrations in old and rare books are often different from modern works. Also, books may not be selected because the physical condition is so fragile that the book may not be able to withstand even occasional use. Unless the item is truly exceptional or it fills a long-standing gap in the collection, most curators will not select an item that requires restoration in order for it to be used. Thus, if the item is not restored by a dealer, a more and more common practice, it may not find a place in a rare book collection in the health sciences.

Price

Is the price a fair one? Prices of rare books are generally high and great care should be exercised to determine whether the offer price is appropriate.

This can be done by checking other dealer catalogs, examining auction records, or consulting with other trusted librarians, private collectors, and dealers.

Research Value of the Artifact over Content

What distinguishes this copy from others, including one which may already be in the collection? A copy with margin annotations by a famous person may make an otherwise commonplace book substantially more important than the original. Special bindings and illustrations too may be of interest, as well as the works of particular publishers.

Provenance

Where has this copy been? Who has owned it? The previous ownership of a particular copy may enhance its value, but rarely its content unless some previous owner made annotations. Because of the large number of copies on the market that have been deaccessioned from other libraries, it is prudent to determine the conditions of the deaccessioning if at all possible. This is particularly important to avoid the purchase of stolen property.

The Subject in Context

Has the discipline changed over time? How? The perception and importance of scientific and medical specialties changes over time. General chemistry in the eighteenth century, for example, is considered core medicine and works in this subject would be highly desirable for some medical rare book collections. Modern day chemistry books, however, are generally considered to be peripheral to core medicine and would not be collected because of changed perceptions of the discipline.

Format

Is the format appropriate for the collection? Are other items of this type already included in the collection? Does the staff expertise to handle the format reside in the staff? Ephemera, manuscripts, artifacts, and microforms may each find a place in a rare book collection as a complement to other materials in the collection. They may also comprise the major part or focus of a special collection. Browsing Tunis's *A Directory of History of Medicine Collections* [34] provides a picture of how prominently formats other than books figure in rare book and history of medicine collections.

Selection Sources

A principal source for information about historical books and important articles in the health sciences is *Morton's Medical Bibliography* [35]. This classic, now in its fifth edition, is considered to be the authority by most curators and rare book librarians in the health sciences. It can be useful in determining which books in specific disciplines are important, in developing desiderata lists, in appraising collections and individual items, and in identifying specialized subject, period, and author bibliographies. *Thornton's Medical Books, Libraries and Collectors* [36] and Corsi's *Information Sources in the History of Medicine and Science* [37] are two additional important source books.

Available items come to the attention of the librarian in different ways, often through a rare book dealer catalog or a notice from the dealer directly to the library. These catalogs and notices frequently have extensive annotations describing the importance of the work itself and the copy in hand. Because these catalogs list single copies, however, speed is of the essence in collection development.

There is a small but very active network of such dealers who make it their business to know the subjects and interests of historical collections. Desiderata lists, or lists of desired items, are commonplace among rare book libraries in all subject disciplines. These lists contain titles which have been determined to be important to an existing collection and the library has determined that it wishes at least to consider purchasing a copy whenever one comes on the market. Such lists are shared with trusted dealers who will keep an eye out for a copy. Auctions are another source for rare medical books, but few librarians attend on their own, preferring to work with a rare book dealer who bids for the library.

References

1. Morse DH, Richards DT. Collection development policies for health sciences libraries. Chicago: Medical Library Association, 1992. (MLA DocKit no. 3).

2. Roper FW, Boorkman JA. Introduction to reference sources in the health sciences. 3rd ed. Metuchen, NJ: Medical Library Association and Scarecrow Press, 1994.

3. Brown JF, Hannigan GG. Microcomputers and reference service. In: Wood MS, ed. Reference and information services in health sciences libraries. Metuchen, NJ: Medical Library Association and Scarecrow Press, 1994. (Current practice in health sciences librarianship, v. 1).

4. Futrelle DP, Curtis JA. Audiovisual, microcomputer, and multimedia reference sources. In: Roper FW, Boorkman JA. Introduction to reference sources in the health sciences. 3rd ed. Metuchen, NJ: Medical Library Association and Scarecrow Press, 1994:173-201.

5. Ibid., 173.

6. Ibid., 174.

7. Ibid., 178.

8. Ibid., 178-89.

9. National Library of Medicine. AVLINE (AudioVisuals OnLINE). Bethesda, MD: National Library of Medicine, 1975-

10. National Library of Medicine. National Library of Medicine audiovisuals catalog. Bethesda, MD: National Library of Medicine, 1977-93.

11. National Information Center for Educational Media. A-V Online. Albuquerque, NM: Access Innovations, 1964-

12. Educational film & video locator. 4th ed. New York: Bowker, 1990.

13. Futrelle, op. cit., 184.

14. The video source book. 13th ed. Detroit: Gale Research, 1992.

15. Film & videofinder. 4th ed. Medford, NJ: Plexus, 1995.

16. Audiovisual & compact disc finder. 3rd ed. Medford, NJ: Plexus, 1993.

17. Filmstrip & slide set finder. Albuquerque, NM: NICEM, 1990.

18. AV market place. New Providence, NJ: Bowker, 1969-

19. Index to AV producers & distributors. 9th ed. Albuquerque, NM: NICEM, 1990.

20. Media profiles: the health sciences edition. West Park, NY: Olympic Media Information, 1984-

21. Health media review index, 1984-86. Metuchen, NJ: Scarecrow Press, 1988.

22. Health reference center. Foster City, CA: Information Access, 1993- .

23. Kernaghan SG, Giloth BE. Consumer health information: managing hospital-based centers. Chicago: Hospital Research and Educational Trust, American Hospital Association, 1992.

24. Rees A, ed. The consumer health information source book. 4th ed. Phoenix, AZ: Oryx Press, 1994.

25. Kernaghan, op. cit., 40-1.

26. Rees, op. cit.

27. Rees A, ed. Consumer health USA: essential information from the Federal Health Network. Phoenix, AZ: Oryx Press, 1995.

28. Mitcham C, Williams WF, eds. The best in science, technology and medicine. New Providence, NJ: Bowker, 1994:309-410. (The reader's adviser, 14th ed., v. 5).

29. Overmier J. Rare books and special collections. Presentation at the MLA Postconference on Collection Development in Health Sciences Libraries, New York, NY, May, 1985.

30. Ibid.

31. Zinn NW. Special collections: history of health science collections, oral history, archives, and manuscripts. In: Darling L, Bishop D, Colaianni LA, eds. Handbook of medical library practice. 4th ed. v. 3. Chicago: Medical Library Association, 1988:472.

32. Ibid., 469-572.

33. Kubinec J, Richards DT. Reference collections in the history of the health sciences: recommendations for policy statements. Presentation at the 84th Annual Meeting of the Medical Library Association, Denver, CO, May 31, 1984.

34. Tunis E. A directory of history of medicine collections. 4th ed. Bethesda, MD: National Library of Medicine, 1993.

35. Norman JM, ed. Morton's medical bibliography: an annotated check-list of texts illustrating the history of medicine (Garrison and Morton). 5th ed. Aldershot, Harts: Scolar Press, 1991.

36. Besson A, ed. Thornton's medical books, libraries and collectors: a study of bibliography and the book trade in relation to the medical sciences. 3rd rev. ed. Brookfield VT: Gower, 1990.

37. Corsi P, Weindling P, eds. Information sources in the history of medicine and science. London: Butterworth, 1983.

8

Budgeting for Collection Development

"At its heart collection management is, indeed, economic. It is the allocation of resources that are severely limited relative to perceived need."

Dennis P. Carrigan

Budgeting is an integral part of collection development. Decisions regarding what to acquire, which mode of access to provide, and what to preserve are all dependent on, and limited by, available funds. Choices must be made within the library's financial environment.

As funding sources shrink, the budgeting function of collection development assumes greater importance. Technology consumes a growing portion of library budgets. All health sciences libraries depend on computer access to medical information, and academic health sciences libraries and larger hospital libraries rely heavily on automation, both for public services and for support operations. All depend on computer access to external resources. In addition, for the last decade price increases for scientific publications have outpaced most budgets. Budget management becomes critical.

The complexity of a library's collection budget will be influenced by numerous factors: the size of the budget, the number of different sources of funds, requirements imposed by the institution's financial offices, and the organization of selecting responsibilities. In most cases, the library director has some flexibility within an institutionally mandated budget structure, and can subdivide the collection budget in response to the library's needs.

Scope of Collection Budget

Deciding what should be encompassed by the collection budget is not as obvious as it sounds. Books and journals, certainly. Audiovisuals, surely. Microforms, of course. CD-ROMs and floppy disks and electronic resources loaded on library-owned equipment, yes—when they contain subject-related content. But what about applications software: word processing, statistical packages, or another step further removed, operating systems, utilities, menu and use-tracking programs, and other systems software? Perhaps not, but what if they also include subject content? The steady advancement of computer technology erases previously neat boundaries and challenges libraries to think about information resources in new ways. Assuming that a basic collection development budget includes major categories for books and journals, some additional categories are discussed in the following sections.

Electronic Databases

As we move beyond stand-alone electronic resources accessible within the library, or even by remote access to the library's local area network, deciding what constitutes "collection" becomes more and more problematic. Should the lease of an institutionally mounted subset of MEDLINE be defined as a collection cost? Even when funding comes from sources beyond the library's regular budget (institutionally supported, user fees, or other means), to add the lease or purchase of a major database is likely to enlarge the collection budget substantially. What if the library belongs to a university system or a multi-institution consortium which acquires and mounts the database at one site, with links throughout the campus or even among multiple campuses, and system costs are shared? When does remote access become local collection? Is only the cost of the database itself considered a collection cost, ignoring the cost of support hardware, software, and telecommunications? Increasingly, these costs cannot be separated. There is no single recommended way to handle budgeting for these resources, but many libraries are incorporating costs for information access into the collection budget. Many collection budgets are evolving into information access budgets.

Remote Online Access

Traditionally, online charges to access remote databases have not been considered collection costs, although functionally, databases such as

MEDLINE or PsychINFO are the equivalent of a published index. Because vendor charges were for access, not for the database itself, and because libraries have often passed on these charges to the user, database access costs have typically been considered separately from collections. However, libraries that view access to information in a more comprehensive sense may well include database access as a collection cost.

Interlibrary Loan or Document Delivery

Should the cost of access to materials not owned by the library be considered a collection cost? Some libraries incorporate interlibrary loan costs, primarily the direct loan charges and copyright fees, and costs for using commercial document delivery services as collection costs. One can argue that it doesn't matter where the material is located as long as the user gets it easily and at the time it is needed. With improved telefacsimile quality and a growing ability to transmit text electronically through national networks like the Internet, obtaining materials from other libraries will be a more acceptable substitute for local ownership. The judgment about what to acquire locally and what to obtain on demand will be more consistently an economic and copyright decision, as the convenience and quality factors will be minimized if not eliminated. The cost of acquiring a document, then, whether it is a single article delivered directly to a requester or a book or journal placed in the library, is an information cost, and in a sense, a collection cost.

Electronic Primary Materials

Electronic journals accessed online from a remote source raise additional questions. They are journals and therefore "collection," and they are subscribed to as if owned, but they are neither owned nor controlled by the subscriber. The initial model, exemplified by the *Online Journal of Current Clinical Trials,* includes use costs similar to those for online current databases. Distribution of electronic journals may also be based on the individual transaction, with charges for each use of an article. If funding comes from the library's budget these costs may be designated as collection costs.

Because the publication format is electronic rather than paper or another more traditional medium is not a reason to exclude such resources from the collection budget. The costs of the primary content, if not the associated equipment and software, certainly belong. However, questions raised by electronic formats and access costs can be difficult to answer. The best advice is to refrain from too rigid a definition of what constitutes the collection and to keep at the forefront the concept that access to information is the primary goal. Budgets, along with librarians, will have to be flexible.

Binding and Preservation

Preservation costs, in part or totally, may be considered part of the collection budget. Routine expenses such as binding may be included as collection costs, although they should be separated from initial book purchase or subscription costs. If the library acquires backup copies of journals on microform or purchases microform to substitute for paper copy in order to conserve space, these costs should also be accounted for in the collection budget. Repairs and more extensive preservation activities are normally handled outside the regular collection budget, although they can certainly be justified as a collection cost. Costs of supplies, such as labels, security devices, and book pockets are generally not accounted for within the collection budget.

Staff Resources

Materials acquired for staff use may be included in the collection budget or the library may choose to budget for them separately as an operations cost. Should dictionaries, manuals, cataloging tools, and database search guides used solely by the staff be charged to collection costs? They may be cataloged for the sake of inventory and location, but they are questionably part of the collection.

Most libraries subscribe to selected professional library journals and purchase occasional books related to library or management issues. Larger health sciences libraries, especially if not located on a general university campus, may maintain a substantial collection for the staff. Should these materials be budgeted for as part of the library's general collection? If the numbers and dollar amounts are small, it probably doesn't make much difference. Because the library staff, regardless of their rank and title within the institution, constitute a legitimate user group for the library, their professional needs should not be ignored, any more than should those of biochemistry faculty or orthopedics residents. Library administration is as appropriate for the collection as is health care administration; health sciences librarianship should be in scope for any health sciences library. While a substantial professional collection may argue for a separate allocation and budget line, it nevertheless belongs within the library's collection budget.

Methods of Allocation

The library's collection budget pie can be sliced in different ways, although the library director may not always have the freedom to select the method used. The following section discusses the advantages and disadvantages of the most common methods of allocation which include by discipline, department, type of material, and location.

By Discipline

Dividing funds by discipline may be considered when selection responsibilities are distributed among several selectors by subject area. For example, one librarian may select material in pediatrics, obstetrics and gynecology, and nursing; another may be responsible for biochemistry, virology, and neurosciences; and a third for public health and hospital administration.

Advantages

1. **Takes into account differences in cost and publishing output by discipline.** When funds are allocated by subject, the difference in cost for different subject areas must be accounted for. In 1995, the average cost of a biochemistry journal was $999; the average cost of a nursing journal was $110. These are extremes, but they make the point that allocations must be based on current costs for materials in the particular subject area. Unless the library is able to maintain comprehensive collections and finds that local costs closely reflect the national averages calculated by vendors, internal allocations should be based on the library's actual costs. Disciplines differ in the amount of literature published, as well as in the relative importance of books, journals, and other materials. New or expanding fields will see greater publication output than those with a more stable knowledge base or narrow focus.

   If done skillfully and carefully, allocating funds based on cost of materials and expected output in different disciplines provides some assurance of balance among subjects that, according to policy, are collected at the same depth. By planning the distribution of spending, all subject areas are covered to a predetermined amount.

2. **Encourages cost analysis and collection assessment.** Allocations by subject require the collection manager or the selector to examine the cost of materials by discipline. This process gives the selector as well as the manager, and in some cases they may be the same indi-

vidual, a more detailed understanding of publishing output and cost of materials in different subjects. With a specific amount of money to spend on anesthesiology, a selector will be prompted to review all the anesthesiology journals to determine that the most needed titles are acquired or to compare several textbooks and decide on the most useful.

3. **Easier to control spending.** If the library uses multiple selectors, there will be multiple eyes on the collection budget. Limits have been preset and each selector must control purchases accordingly.

4. **Delegates responsibility to individual selectors and provides information for performance reviews.** If selection responsibilities are distributed, each selector may have funds assigned to the specific disciplines for which that selector is responsible. This forces the selector to take into account the cost of materials and the comparative value of different publications in the same subject area. A selector who has only so much to spend is more likely to exercise critical thinking than if someone else is responsible for managing the dollars.

5. **Provides useful data.** Information about the amount of money a library spends on collections in specific disciplines is often requested by accrediting bodies. They use these data as a measure of how well the library is supporting residency or other health training programs.

Disadvantages

1. **Difficult to define subjects.** Deciding how specific the categories should be can be problematic. Should neurology and neurosciences be separate funds? Should each of the internal medicine specialties receive an allocation: cardiology, oncology, rheumatology, allergy? Should microbiology and virology be together? What about genetics, molecular biology, and biotechnology? How should the relevant social sciences be handled? Should materials on eye surgery come out of the allocation for surgery or for ophthalmology? Increasingly medical research is interdisciplinary; what should be done with pediatric orthopedics, immunotoxicology, or neuropsychopharmacology? Should specialties like sports medicine, women's health, and bioethics be separate categories, even if the number of materials published or acquired is small?

2. **Hard to achieve balance in assignments.** Disciplines vary greatly in the amount of literature published and this can make spreading the workload evenly among selectors troublesome.

3. **Cumbersome to administer.** Keeping track of allocations and spending by multiple discipline incurs costs in administrative time, even with automated accounting. Someone has to determine the subject area to which a purchase or subscription will be assigned. Someone has to collect and analyze the data to determine how the funds will be distributed by subject. Someone has to monitor each subject area during the year and determine when adjustments in spending are required.
4. **Less flexible.** By assigning collection funds to specific subjects, a decision process and mechanism are required to shift funds from one subject to another or to make special purchases that overlap more than one area. If funds for dentistry are more than adequate, but microbiology is short and selectors agree to purchase some microbiology materials with the dentistry allocation, then the data on expenditures and number of materials purchased on each of those subjects will be inaccurate unless special records are kept.
5. **May lead to complacency.** Users and library staff alike may assume that because the funds are divided by subject, each area will be adequately covered. If the distribution of funds does not match the publication output and needs, important purchases may not be made.

While prevalent in academic libraries where very broad divisions equivalent in scope to all of medicine are used, allocation by discipline in health sciences libraries is less common. In many cases the disadvantages outweigh the benefits.

By Department

Allocating funds by department or other institutional unit differs in some respects from allocating by discipline, although there are obvious similarities. In addition to the advantages and disadvantages outlined for division by subject, budgeting by department deserves special comment, both in terms of benefits and disadvantages.

Advantages

1. **Fewer allocation categories.** The number of departments in an institution is finite and can be named. It is usually clear who has appointments in the department of physiology, or who is in physical therapy. In some cases, allocations may be for even broader units, such as the school of nursing, college of pharmacy, and the like.

2. **Easier to link faculty or clinical staff representatives with the library.** If the library has a formal liaison program in which department representatives assist the library with collection decisions, a budget allocation clearly identified with the area they represent will make budget-related decisions more understandable and in some cases more defendable to them. If they accept the basic distribution, then decisions necessary to stay within the department allocation do not pit departments or disciplines against each other.
3. **Provides accountability to departments.** Tracking expenditures for materials needed for departmental clinical or research activities may be useful in developing budget requests for the library. Individual departments may support funding requests that are directly related to their needs.
4. **Encourages interdepartmental cooperation.** In times of budget austerity, departments may be willing to negotiate reallocation of funds or support shared funding for interdisciplinary materials. Predetermined allocations provide a framework for cooperation of this type.

Disadvantages

1. **Difficult to define.** Despite the foregoing statement that the number of departments will be limited and obvious, most health science institutions, whether they are health professional schools or hospitals, or combinations of the two, are complex and not neatly organized. What should be done with a specialized diabetes institute, a burn unit, a biotechnology center? Not only may there be more categories than if strict disciplinary subdivisions are used but there will be more overlap among them. Additionally, materials for students in health professional education programs may be difficult to allocate when funds are distributed by specialty department.
2. **More proprietary interest.** If departments or other clinical or research units recognize that funds have been earmarked to cover their particular needs, using those funds to purchase materials that have significant or even predominant use by other departments can create conflict. Similarly the department may view allocated funds as "theirs" and dictate to the library how the funds are to be spent. If material on drug abuse is purchased for pharmacy but is heavily used by medical and nursing students and the social work department, the college of pharmacy may argue that not all the cost should come from "their" allocation. Delicate negotiations must then ensue. The potential for negative political consequences of such an approach may outweigh any advantages.

3. Uneven participation. If departments are expected to play an active role in selection, the library must be vigilant to see that inequities don't result from some departments being more vocal or aggressive than others. Normally the library should not rely on individual users to initiate purchase suggestions, although they may turn to them for evaluation or approval.

By Type of Material

Many health sciences libraries divide their collection budgets by type of material—commonly journals, books, electronic resources, audiovisual materials, and occasionally other categories. This approach has advantages over the subject allocations as well as disadvantages.

Advantages

1. **Easy to define.** There are relatively few difficulties in deciding which publications are journals and which are audiovisuals. The budget can be quite simple, divided only by major categories, or it can be further subdivided. Monographic series on standing order may be budgeted separately from journals or books. A budget category may be established for new journals. Computer-based resources such as CD-ROMs and diskettes may be placed in a separate budget category or combined with other formats.
2. **Separates materials that are priced and paid for in different ways.** Vendor costs also differ. Journal subscriptions are paid for annually or for multiple years and often incur a vendor service charge. Firm prices may not be known until after the budget has been set and subscription commitments have been made. Preliminary subscription costs may be increased later with added charges. Journal prices are also heavily affected by fluctuations in foreign currency exchange rates. Once the subscriptions are established for the year, little manipulation of the budget is possible.

   Because budgeting is handled differently for ongoing subscriptions and for single item purchases and prices per title or per item differ greatly for various media, separating them in the budget is almost necessary for effective management.

Disadvantages

1. **Overemphasis on format.** One could argue that budgeting by type of material allows the collection to be driven by format, resulting in

the protection of journal subscriptions over book purchases, even in disciplines where book publication is more significant. Careful analysis of needs and reassessment of allocations each year should assure proper balance.

2. **Does not account for discipline-related costs.** Most libraries use some form of automation for ordering, cataloging, and financial operations. Even if the collection budget is allocated by type of material, subscriptions and one-time purchases can usually be coded by subject. With a well-designed integrated library system, data should be easily obtained from subject coded fields linked with payment records. Even if the local library system cannot produce data on cost by subject, serial and book vendors can usually provide it for their clients. These methods can overcome some of the disadvantages of not allocating collection funds by discipline.

Type of material and subject area can be combined and for special purposes it may make sense to do this. If the library serves more than one professional school, a separate allocation, say for nursing or public health, may be needed both for practical and political reasons. Each of these budgets may then be subdivided by type of material or the budget organization could also be reversed, with book and journal allocations subdivided by discipline.

By Location

Under some circumstances the budget may be divided by location of materials. This approach can be useful for setting aside funds for special purposes: reference or reserve collections, rare books departments, off-campus satellite collections, or branch libraries.

In most cases, the allocations for separate locations will be in addition to a basic budget division by discipline or type of material. It is a way of assuring a certain level of support for special needs. A library may wish to commit a certain amount of money to a leisure reading collection (less common in times of tight budgets) or to a patient education reading area. Having a separate allocation both encourages a certain level of spending and places a cap on it. In addition, it provides accountability to the organization and demonstrates library support for institutional programs.

Current practice in health sciences libraries is to separate funds by format and sometimes by broad programs, such as nursing or medicine [1]. Widespread use of automated systems to track information and manipulate data on a variety of variables related to expenditures and materials has reduced the need for a highly structured budget. Increased accountability, however, suggests that whatever allocation mechanism is used, the library should make sure it provides sufficient data to be responsive to institutional administrators.

Making Allocation Decisions

Distributing Funds

If the collection budget is divided into categories, whether they are for different subject areas, different departments, various types of collections, or different types of material—or combinations of these factors—decisions about distributing the funds to these categories must be made.

Allocating by discipline or department requires substantial knowledge of publications and costs within the different fields, as well as an understanding of the institutional needs in each area. Comparative data on the number of books and journals published and average costs will be needed to determine the relative proportion of the budget that should be assigned to each topic. Past practice can sometimes be used as a guide, if there is general satisfaction that the collection is balanced and adequately fulfills current needs. For books, the collection's distribution by classification may be used to determine proportion by subject, adjusted by differences in average price per book. If this method is used, only the past few years should be used, as needs change over time. Libraries that purchase most of their books through a single medical bookseller should also be able to obtain this information from the vendor.

If journal allocations are also made by subject, the number of journals that meet selection criteria and their average prices can form the base for distributing the funds. Once set, however, the distribution may not vary substantially from year to year, although it should be reviewed periodically. While some journals will cease or be canceled and new titles will be added, the main change factor will be price.

One of the biggest concerns of academic and scientific libraries, including health sciences, is the proportion of their collection budget devoted to serials. Once a subscription is established, the funds are locked up, at least for the year, and libraries are notoriously reluctant to discontinue long-standing subscriptions. Multiyear subscriptions or prepayment arrangements extend the commitment further. While most standing orders for book series can be canceled at any time, some other continuing orders may be more difficult to discontinue on short notice. If the library has committed a high proportion of its budget to subscriptions, that not only reduces the ability to purchase other materials when needed, but results in very little flexibility to adjust spending if price increases turn out to be higher than anticipated. If most funds are committed, there is no buffer to absorb unforeseen increases. Each library must analyze its own needs for different types of materials, guided by its collection policy, and judge the degree of risk it can reasonably assume in making financial commitments. A general recommendation is to establish a ceiling of 85% of the budget devoted to serials. In bad times, continuing orders for series or new editions can be canceled in favor of individual purchase decisions.

Using Formulas

Formulas for determining the size and distribution of the collection budget are sometimes used in academic libraries [2-4]. Most often formulas are applied to book purchases; in a survey of academic libraries, Budd found only 10% used allocation formulas for serials [5]. Formulas in academic libraries are often based on the number of students at different levels, credit hours, or number of faculty. Other formulas may account for differences in average cost of materials by discipline, the relative emphasis on periodical and book literature, or use of collections. One method that takes into account both use and relative size of collections calculates the amount of collection use in each subject compared to the total collection use for a given time period and divides this percentage by the percentage of the total collection each subject represents. The resultant "proportional use statistic" may then be used to determine the allocation for books [6].

The literature on formulas can be found in articles and books on collection development in academic libraries. The validity of formulas has been debated over the years. As critics point out, formulas do not inherently offer greater accountability, although they may promote consistency over time. "The difficulties of any formulaic approach lie in determining the elements to be measured and then in measuring them accurately" [7]. In the words of Brownson, "Accountability need not be by allocation; allocation need not be by subject; subject allocation need not be by formula" [8]; he then goes on to propose yet another formula based on an index of factors relating to collection strength, need (use), and research activities and tied to the collection policy.

Formulas may also be more difficult to apply when budgets are severely limited, arguing against developing complex methods of determining allocations.

Access to information, rapid document delivery, co-operative efforts to rationalize collection purchases between institutions, can have more profound results in meeting immediate user demands than wasting a great deal of effort attempting to divide an inadequate collection budget amongst a variety of disciplines [9].

In addition to some of the elements suggested by academic libraries, health sciences libraries might consider such factors as the most common discharge diagnoses in the hospital, the disciplines in which the institution supports residency programs, and centers of research emphasis. These factors should, and in fact very often do, determine the collection emphasis, but few libraries have determined numerical weightings and translated these into dollar figures or percentages for fund distribution. Formulas obviously only address those factors that can be quantified. Other factors may enter into decision making, such as historical precedent or importance or uniqueness of specific programs.

Approval Plans

When an approval plan is used to acquire books that match a given profile by subject and publisher, expenditures should be estimated annually. For an approval plan to be cost- effective for the vendor as well as the receiving library, the return rate for rejected material should be minimized. If the library's expenditures for books must be reduced and the approval plan is likely to be significantly affected, the profile should be reviewed and altered, as needed, to avoid excessive returns for budgetary reasons alone. Expenditures for books on approval plans should be tracked to determine what percentage of the total book budget they consume. This information will aid in budget decisions for the following year.

Reserve Funds

Although not a common practice when budgets are lean, a contingency fund may be established by large libraries with extensive budgets. This fund is not specifically allocated by subject or type of material and may be used if journal prices or other costs exceed the budgeted amount, or for special purchases at the end of the year. While helpful for dealing with the uncertainties of journal subscription costs, most libraries will not have the luxury of setting aside reserve funds.

Cost Analysis

Cost of materials has been mentioned repeatedly in discussing how the collection budget may be allocated. The collection manager should make use of multiple sources in assessing costs.

Local Information

The best place to start is at home, examining the cost of materials actually acquired by the library, including trends over time. There are numerous ways to examine the costs. Simple spreadsheet software may be used if the library doesn't have an automated system or if its automated system isn't able to track costs according to the desired variables, such as subject, publisher, and type of material. One of the advantages of using a major vendor for books and journals is the data the vendor is able to provide regarding cost trends, both nationwide and specific to the customer library. Often these reports are offered as a standard benefit of the subscription service or approval plan; at additional cost a library may also request customized reports for particular purposes.

Published Sources of Data

The *Bowker Annual Library and Book Trade Almanac* [10] publishes reports on publishing output and average prices for books and journals based primarily on vendor data. Although useful for a general picture of the publishing industry and to place the more specific information about health sciences materials in a broader context, these sources are too broad to be used for developing the library's local budget. The *Bowker Annual* data are two years old and would be useful only for trend analysis or historical information. Somewhat more specific are the price index of U.S. periodicals and serial services (published by the American Library Association in *Library Journal* for the Association for Library Collections and Technical Services [ALCTS] Library Materials Price Index Committee [11]) and the report on average prices of journals in major indexes in *Serials Review.* Published regularly for many years, these articles represent critical reviews of data from major periodical vendors (the Faxon and EBSCO companies). Of particular value is the cost analysis of *Index Medicus* journals reported annually in *Serials Review* [12-13]. These analyses measure price changes (primarily increases) against a predetermined index year.

For small health sciences libraries, the price analysis of medical books and journals included in the introduction to the Brandon/ Hill list for small medical libraries, published in the *Bulletin of the Medical Library Association* in alternate years, may be especially useful, both in developing and justifying a collection budget [14]. Price data compiled for specific subject areas may be found in library or specialty publications. Brandon and Hill publish information biennially on nursing collections with their core list in *Nursing Outlook* [15] and for allied health in the *Bulletin of the Medical Library Association* [16]. An analysis of veterinary medicine journals is published annually in *The Serials Librarian* [17]. The relative publishing output for broad health sciences subjects appears in Table 1-1.

Making Predictions

Predicting costs is necessary for responsible budgeting and long-range planning. On the other hand, accurate predictions are impossible. The crystal ball must encompass publishing trends, the consumer price index, the cost of paper, publisher pricing policies, the higher education index, the cost of oil, postal rates, foreign currency exchange rates, labor strikes, tax structure, publisher mergers, copyright laws, international conflict, and general economic health both in the United States and the rest of the world. Many factors, in addition to the profit motive, may cause a publisher to increase subscription prices (journal size, method of delivery, circulation, currency exchange) [18]. Predicting the future based on the past is the most common approach, although any of the many influencing factors can change the picture. Over the past two decades, however, the trend has been steadily upward, with cost of materials increasing at rates far higher than those included in either the general consumer price index or the higher education index. Publications in the sciences, including medicine, have seen the greatest increases.

While economic forecasting is a specialized career for which few library managers are trained, some techniques for making projections may be borrowed from this field. Perhaps the most useful is regression analysis, which under certain circumstances can discern trends that may be projected into the future. Its reliability depends on the existence of a fairly steady trend and relatively constant changes from year to year. There must be an underlying pattern into which the annual data fit.

If future costs are being predicted on the basis of a sample of past costs, care must be taken to use an adequate sample size. Extreme variations in prices, especially for journals and electronic resources, make accurate sampling difficult. While long-range estimates may seem futile, short-range predictions, shaky though they may be, must be built into budget planning. In the past, publishers have not been very forthcoming regarding their pricing, even for the coming year. Book and journal vendors may often be the best source for educated guesswork. They attempt to keep up not only with publishers' policies, but with foreign exchange rates and other factors that may affect pricing.

Sources of Funds

Institutional Funds

Because maintaining the collection is considered one of its core functions, the library's regular budget allocated by the institution will support most of the expenditures for collections. In many cases, the budget approved by the administration to which the library reports will specify the amount allocated for collections, and may even indicate how much will be designated for journals, books, or other types of materials. In other institutions, the library receives a single allocation, to be distributed as the library administration determines. While the latter offers the greatest flexibility, it may also mean that the collection budget receives no special protection by the institution. Some institutions have special sources for one-time funds that may be requested or applied for to supplement the regular budget.

Indirect Cost Recovery

Some research grant guidelines allow investigators to include the cost of library materials needed to support their research project. In addition, most federal grants include indirect costs, at a percentage negotiated by the institution, which frequently include cost factors for library services. Because many fingers attempt to get into this pie, from the state level down to the individual researcher, few libraries successfully recover any of these monies, but it is a resource that may be tapped in some institutions. The attempt should at least be made.

Donations

Gifts related to collections may be of two types: money or actual publications. Issues related to donated materials are discussed in Chapter 5, Selection: Journals and Books. As noted, they can be a mixed blessing, but under certain circumstances may be a welcome supplement, especially for materials not otherwise available.

Monetary gifts applicable to collections, unless complicated by too many restrictions, are usually accepted gladly. When there is a large user base or a supportive community a program to encourage donations as memorials or honors can bring in substantial funds. There are associated costs for acknowledgments, book plates, and record-keeping, but with some effort these costs can be minimized. An active Friends group can both promote such a program and may in some cases handle paperwork. Hospital auxiliaries, medical staff associations, alumni, and even parents or spouse groups may be potential sources of gift funds. Some donors will respond better to the idea that their gift will be used for enhancement of the collections—for special materials that would not be encompassed by the library's regular budget—rather than by a more general appeal for budget relief, which implies that the institution is inadequately supporting the library.

Although tempting during times of budget reductions and price increases, relying on faculty or others to donate journals is rarely satisfactory [19]. Another approach to obtain help with subscription costs in which the subscription remains under the library's control is an "adopt a journal" program. Such a program seeks sponsors for individual journals subscribed to by the library; however, takers for expensive journals may be hard to find.

Endowments

Endowments, a special form of gift, can provide long-term support for collections. Significant donors may be encouraged to extend their dollars by setting up an endowment fund from which purchases may be made in their name or in memory of someone. If endowment funds are to be used for special collections, the library should consider suggesting that the donor include processing and preservation costs as well as purchase of publications. Interest from large gifts may provide ongoing funds for many years. The amount of accrued interest will vary according to institutional investment practices and interest rates. Unless restricted by the donor, substantial endowments can provide a safety net for the library. Often, however, donors may prefer to designate an endowment for special purchases or rare books, which can allow a library to build up important research collections that would not otherwise be possible.

Exchanges

If a library's parent institution publishes a medical journal, book series, or other ongoing publication that might be of interest to another institution which issues a journal the library desires, an exchange arrangement may be possible. Such arrangements are particularly useful for obtaining foreign publications, especially when there is difficulty with currency exchange. These opportunities are not common in medical institutions and exchange programs do not have a major effect on collection development or budgets in health sciences libraries.

Fund Raising

Opportunities to raise funds for the library collections are often over-looked. Events such as the ongoing or periodic sale of duplicates or un-needed gift publications, or book sales of donated books are common methods. The ability to sell duplicates or materials weeded from the library's collection may be limited by institutional or state restrictions on disposal of property. Ideas for fund raising events are often published in library periodicals and in the newsletter of the *Friends of Libraries U.S.A.* [20].

Grants for special purposes, especially from local foundations or institutions, should also be considered.

Budget Preparation

Budget requests should be based on defined needs, accurate data, and informed predictions.

Determining Needs

The first step in preparing a collection budget request is to determine needs for the next funding period. Not all elements within the budget are equally important in predicting future needs. The manager should select which categories to use in making budget projections. Which factors will influence needs most? Cost increases, number of publications, new media, interlibrary borrowing transactions, and library use are examples. Anticipate new programs or changes in direction for teaching, clinical services, and research activities. Match the budget emphasis with institutional priorities.

Presenting the Budget

Most institutions will have some type of formal budget process in which the library participates, but the format and content requirements will vary widely from institution to institution. In spite of this variation, several general principles apply.

1. *Know the audience.* A budget request is generally a written document, but this principle holds true for oral presentations as well. Who makes the budget decisions? Is this the same person who receives the request? If not, does the request have to be understood, supported, and defended by someone else at a higher level in the organization? Who really has to be convinced that the request is justified? The budget should be presented with the critical individuals in mind—whether it is the director's immediate boss or administrators at a higher level: a vice president, a hospital director, or a library board. Woe to the library whose budget request goes directly to a financial officer!

2. *Fit the document or presentation to the critical audience.* What are their highest priorities? If possible demonstrate where the library supports or complements those programs. What are their chief concerns? Acknowledge these issues and take them into account. Try to understand their viewpoint and emphasize functions whose value will be obvious and describe needs in language that is understandable to them. A budget request may be thought of as a sales presentation. This is not to suggest that it should be manipulative or misleading, but to indicate the importance of connecting the library's needs to the institutional context and presenting them in a way that will be meaningful and convincing to the decision makers.

3. *Be concise.* Again, know your audience. Does the administrator typically like lots of detail or prefer a general statement and summary? Don't create a comprehensive explanation of every need, when all the administrator wants is a brief outline and total amount. If you report to a numbers person, emphasize numbers. If you report to a concept person, do not overwhelm with figures. A useful approach in many cases is to present a clear one-page summary giving the highlights and total figures, followed by greater detail for those who need or want it. Do not bore the reader or the audience.

4. *Follow directions.* If the institution specifies a format for budget requests, present the information in the requested manner, even if you prefer another form of presentation. This is not the time to be innovative. Even if the library is not required to follow the same format as other departments in the organization, it may be advantageous to do so. In some situations this may increase the visibility of the library and place its request on the same footing as other units.

5. *Be credible.* Be sure you understand everything in the budget document and can back it up with reliable information. The derivation of budget figures should be appended, even if not part of the primary document; show your work. Assess alternatives before presenting a request. A budget request should not be viewed as a wish list. Taken more than once, this approach is likely to result in a quick loss of credibility. It is the rare hospital or university that has funds to toss at frivolous or poorly thought-out programs. Do the homework before the test, not after.

6. *Be accurate.* In every group or organization is a bean counter, one who will check the totals and percentages in every column and one who will compare Table 1 with Table 7. Inevitably that person will find the one transposed number or misplaced decimal. Spreadsheets greatly reduce the chance of clerical errors, but this does not mean that vigilance can be relaxed. The numbers must make sense. One error and the entire document becomes suspect. Sloppiness in a budget document is less forgivable than in an annual report.

7. *Be compelling.* A budget presentation is a public relations opportunity for the library. You have the attention of the institution; take advantage of it. Both in a written document and in an oral presentation, selective use of graphics can have a greater impact than words or numbers alone. Easy-to-use graphics programs, whether associated with word processing or spreadsheet software or stand alone, are both a boon and a hazard. Choose only those graphics that clearly illustrate an important point—for example, changes in the degree to which different client groups use library services; or the effect of rising journal prices on the purchasing power of the budget. Overuse of graphics lessens their impact; avoid including them simply because they are easy to produce.

8. *Use comparisons.* Comparisons with other libraries can be very effective to make a point, but should be used sparingly. The peer group selected for comparison should be one that is recognized by the parent institution and should have similar characteristics. However, beware that sometimes these two attributes will conflict.

9. *Be prepared.* Anticipate questions that may be raised or arguments that may be made for not supporting the requested budget. If the argument for interlibrary loan in lieu of purchase for a greater number of journals is made, be ready with cost data and information regarding copyright restrictions if they are appropriate to the question. On the other hand, avoid being overly defensive and be receptive to alternative solutions to budgetary challenges.

Budget Management

A budget document serves multiple purposes. It communicates how resources are allocated and accounts for expenditures. It also demonstrates the rationale for allocation decisions and relates them to institutional needs and priorities. The American Library Association's *Guide to Budget Allocation for Information Resources* suggests the general content for budget documents and steps in the allocation process, as well as criteria for allocation and budgeting tools [21].

The organization of the library's collection budget may take different forms for different purposes. While the official budget may be structured according to fixed categories dictated by the institutional or library administration such as books, journals, or department allocations, different categories may be used in predicting costs and assessing budget needs, while a third grouping might be used in actually presenting the budget request. Automated systems provide the flexibility to analyze, monitor, and report data to accommodate different management needs.

Books, journal subscriptions, and outright purchases of other materials are normally considered capital expenditures—costs for nonconsumable, tangible items owned by the library. Costs to access remote databases, copyright payments, licenses for databases or other electronic resources, and cataloging or interlibrary loan system use charges may be included in the collection budget but fall outside the definition of capital expenses. The structure of the budget document may need to conform to institutional definitions as well as reflect logically related costs.

Redistributing

Once a budget for the library has been approved, it is then the responsibility of the library administration to make the final distribution, unless of course, the library is given no flexibility to do this. In the fortunate event that the full amount requested is received, little or no redistribution will be necessary. On the other hand, when funding does not match the request, decisions will have to be made. A good manager should both anticipate the outcome of the request through continual communication within the institution and be prepared with alternatives to full funding.

In some cases, the needs for collections must be weighed against other library needs. There may be tradeoffs with other budget categories. Within the collection budget, priorities should be clear and guided by the collection development policy.

Monitoring

Establishing a collection budget for the year is only the beginning. It must then be monitored throughout the year, and corrective action taken as needed to stay within the library's allocation. Fiscal policies will differ from institution to institution. Medical school libraries in state universities will be constrained both by university practices and by state requirements. Health sciences libraries in private universities and hospitals will operate under the guidelines for those organizations.

The degree of budget flexibility will vary. The greatest flexibility is achieved when the library director can freely move funds from one budget line to another and can carry over unspent funds from year to year. In many cases, however, this degree of freedom to manage the budget is not permitted. Quite commonly, funds cannot be shifted between fixed categories, such as personnel, capital, and operating funds. If the budget for the collection is approved separately, it may not be possible to shift funds from other parts of the library's budget to supplement the initial allocation. Less commonly, the allocations for designated subdivisions of the collection budget are also fixed. In this case, it might be difficult to use funds allocated to monographs to cover unexpected price increases in journals, or even to spend an anticipated surplus in the allocation for ophthalmology to purchase additional materials in genetics. Funds from endowments, grants, or other sources that are restricted to specific purposes, of course, must be used only for those purposes.

Some fiscal practices, while possibly making business sense to the organization as a whole, cause special problems for collection management in libraries. Some institutions require approval for purchases over a certain amount; some require libraries to use vendors on state contracts; some prohibit prepayments or make them extremely difficult. Health sciences libraries are highly dependent on journals. Subscriptions must be renewed prior to the year of receipt, often without knowing the final price. The inability to carry over funds from one year to the next hampers the manager from reserving funds from the current year to cover anticipated increases the next year and buffering the library's users from precipitous journal cancellations or abrupt cessation of book purchases. The good collection manager will continue to gather information from many sources throughout the year, constantly adjusting projections for the future.

Book and other single item purchases should be made steadily throughout the year, as materials are published or requested. Toward the latter part of the fiscal year, monitoring should be more frequent and more diligent, and adjustments made to speed up or defer purchases. Journal expenditures, on the other hand, will be negligible, except for single purchases such as supplements, replacement volumes, or the occasional title acquired directly from the publisher, until the vendor's annual renewal invoice is received, usually in the fall. At this point, if journals are a separate line in the collection budget, that fund will be depleted and the collection budget will then be largely spent, even though many months may remain in the fiscal year.

The manager must understand the pattern of payment for the library—know when in the year the large invoices are paid, how much of the budget should remain after they are paid, approximately how much to expect in added charges, be aware of special purchases to be made that year, such as expensive cumulative indexes, and if the library has a significant number of multiyear subscriptions, to know when they are due for renewal. Maintaining a comparative spreadsheet or graph, showing expenditures by month for each year, allows the collection manager to judge the health of the budget. If after the major journal invoice has been paid, the journal budget is 93% spent when past history indicates that at that time expenditures are normally only 85% of the year's total, this variation is a flag prompting the fund manager to investigate.

Managing Crises

Textbooks instruct administrators to avoid management by crisis; but it is equally important to learn how to effectively manage crisis when it does occur—an inevitable component of organizational life. With long-range planning, use of predictive techniques, and alertness to changes in external factors, the need for sudden action should be largely preventable. However, the manager also needs on occasion to respond to unexpected circumstances.

When price predictions miss the mark significantly or the institution's budget picture changes suddenly, the collection manager may need to act quickly. The most welcome of these situations is when the library is asked at the last minute to spend a substantial sum in a short period of time—typically funds remaining in an account that can't be carried over and the library is selected as a recipient because it can spend money quickly and because it serves a broad clientele, thus causing the least controversy. If the institution habitually makes these year-end contributions, the library should be prepared by keeping a list of special items that are really needed but cannot be acquired out of the regular allocation. An unexpected windfall from a large gift may cause a brief flurry of decision-making and scrambling to identify appropriate uses, but is usually managed without difficulty. Care should be taken that, however tempting, one-time funds not be used to establish new ongoing commitments, such as journal subscriptions. Such funds might be used to extend renewals in a difficult year, to avert a crisis, with the full realization that this does not solve the problem, but simply buys time to make more rational decisions.

A more dismal crisis is the sudden reduction of the library's budget. This action is generally related to institutional and state budgets and often reflects more global economic health—the region, the nation, even the world. Often, even these situations can be anticipated and the wise manager will be prepared with a general approach and a method for making decisions. Is there a review process in place that can be activated on a larger scale? Are faculty or staff involved in collection development on an ongoing basis or only during times of crisis or reduction? The library may find greater support if its users have a good understanding of the process and criteria for making collection decisions and routinely participate in the process.

Does the library have a clear set of priorities for its collections? In developing a collection policy some attention should be given to how the policy might help guide a collection reduction. Where are the strengths? Where are the weaknesses? Are they reviewed periodically to assure that they still match the current emphasis in patient care or research? None of this will eliminate the occasional need for quick, decisive action, but the result of a budget cut conducted with a clear set of priorities and a rational, participative process will have a less harmful effect on the institution than one conducted capriciously or with only hasty thought.

Communicating

Staying within the budget is essential. Careful management avoids either over or under spending. Equally important is continued communication regarding the budget status and needs. If a collection manager has primary responsibility for the collection budget, the director should receive regular reports and communication regarding expenditures, new and deferred needs, and any new data on costs.

Also, the institutional administrator to whom the library reports should be kept informed. The level of detail and format will vary according to the position and style of the administrator. The best rule to follow is—don't surprise the boss. The library director also has a responsibility to see that those who are responsible for overseeing and monitoring the institutional budget understand where library collection expenditures are unique. In institutions with a fiscal year starting in September or October, it should be made clear that the bulk of the collection budget will be spent in the first few months, at the time that the journal subscriptions are renewed with the vendor. This is the normal pattern, not a cause for alarm. Also, if the fiscal year coincides with the calendar year, the budget will remain largely intact until near the end of the year. If there is good communication between the library and institutional budget officers, these deviations will not cause problems.

References

1. Symposium on fund allocation. Biomed Libr Acq Bull [serial online] 1994 Nov 23, no. 34; Dec 6, no. 35. Available from: University of Southern California, Norris Medical Library, Los Angeles via Internet.

2. McGrath WE, Huntsinger RC, Barber GR. An allocation formula derived from a factor analysis of academic departments. Coll Res Libr 1969 Jan;30 (1):51-62.

3. McGrath WE. A pragmatic book allocation formula for academic and public libraries with a test for its effectiveness. Libr Res Tech Serv 1975 Fall;19(4):356-69.

4. Budd JM. Allocation formulas in the literature: a review. Libr Acq Pract Theory 1991;15(1):95-107.

5. Budd JM, Adams K. Allocation formulas in practice. Libr Acq Pract Theory 1989;13(4):381- 90.

6. Carrigan DP. Improving return on investment: a proposal for allocating the book budget. J Acad Libr 1992 Nov;18(5): 292-7.

7. Martin MS. The allocation of money within the book budget. In: Stueart RD, Miller GB, eds. Collection development in libraries; a treatise. Part A. Greenwich, CT: JAI Press, 1980:35-66.

8. Brownson CW. Modeling library materials expenditure: initial experiments at Arizona State University. Libr Res Tech Serv 1991 Jan;35(1):87-103.

9. Kelly GJ. Using an economic development approach to improve budget forecasting techniques, collection allocation methods, and library budgeting decisions. In: Katz B, ed.Vendors and library acquisitions. Binghamton, NY: Haworth Press, 1991:191-213.

10. Bowker Annual Library and Book Trade Almanac. Annual. New Providence, NJ: R.R. Bowker.

11. Ketcham L, Born K. Projecting the electronic revolution while budgeting for the status quo. 36th annual report: periodical price survey 1996. Libr J 1996 Apr 15;121(7):45-51.

12. Brooke FD Jr, Powell A. EBSCO 1995 serial price projections. Ser Rev 1994 Fall;20(3):850-94.

13. Fortney LM, Basile VA. Index Medicus price study: 1991-1995. Ser Rev 1995 Fall;21(3):47-74.

14. Brandon AN, Hill DR. Selected list of books and journals for the small medical library. Bull Med Libr Assoc 1995 Apr;83(2):151-75.

15. Brandon AN, Hill DR. Selected list of nursing books and journals. Nurs Outlook 1996 Mar/Apr; 44(2):56-66.

16. Brandon AN, Hill DR. Selected list of books and journals in allied health. Bull Med Libr Assoc 1996 Jul;84(3):289-309.

17. Fackler NP. Journals for academic veterinary medical libraries: price increases, 1983-1994. Ser Libr 1995;27(4):41-50.

18. Henderson A. Forecasting changes in periodical prices. Ser Libr 1992;21(4):33-43.

19. Grefsheim SF, Bader SA, Meredith PA. Personal/departmental journal subscriptions: panacea or pandora for a library's journal collection. Bull Med Libr Assoc 1984 Apr;72(2):208-9.

20. Friends of Libraries U.S.A. National Notebook. Quarterly. Chicago: Friends of Libraries USA.

21. Shreeves E, ed. Guide to budget allocation for information resources. Subcommittee on Budget Allocation, Collection Management and Development Committee, Resources Section, Association for Library Collections and Technical Services. Chicago: American Library Association, 1991. (Collection management and development guides, no. 4).

9

Collection Assessment

"Regular, systematic collection assessments are essential to a well-managed collection development program."

Blaine Hall, 1985

"Evaluation of collections has been and is being made constantly. Each time a user finds desired information, and even more so each time he does not, an evaluation of the collection . . . has been vouchsafed. We need not dwell on this, except to note its existence and further to suggest that, whether ill-informed or not, these evaluations are in the long run those that will probably count the most."

David Henige, 1991

Programmatic collection evaluation can be traced to the mid-nineteenth century with Jewett's 1849 comparative analysis of citations in several lists of notable books in international law, chemistry, and anthropology [1]. The lists were compared against holdings of major libraries to substantiate the budget request for the Smithsonian Library, which he directed. Following Jewett, collection evaluations were principally narrative descriptions of the high points of the collection such as the great works of scholarship, medieval authors, and the like. It was not until the 1930s and 1940s that true collection assessment began to emerge. Its principal purpose was to demonstrate the inadequacy of holdings. The most popular method of evaluation in the early part of the twentieth century was comparison of individual holdings to those in a scholarly or "select" bibliography. These bibliographies had the endorsement of major professional associations including ALA. The librarian used the bibliography as an "indirect expert" to make qualitative statements about the utility of the collection. An early and important assessment of the NLM collection was undertaken by Keyes

Metcalf in the 1940s [2]. The report of this survey, financed by the Rocke-
feller Foundation, is an important historical document in the literature of
health sciences librarianship.

The drafting of policy and criteria and the documentation of procedures
for implementing those policies and criteria provide the framework for
developing a collection over time. Collection assessment or evaluation
allows the librarian to examine how well that framework has served and
continues to serve the library and the institution. Collection evaluation
studies can be complex or simple and can be done as projects or integrated
into collection development routines. Data from such studies allow librarians to make adjustments to those routines, and also to enhance practical
routines, such as budget justifications and requests for additional funding
support or for the reallocation of existing funds. These data also allow for
greater assurance in setting collection development priorities and for developing a systematic plan for collection enrichment.

Collection assessment studies themselves are useful in staff education
because these studies require that one become familiar with the literature
of a discipline. This familiarity should result in a greater awareness of the
elements of that literature and lead to more finely honed collection development skills among the librarians in charge of building the collection in a
particular discipline. Results from studies may also be helpful in enhancing
communication between librarian and user, as well as selector-to-selector
communication. The effort establishes a common base for discussion with
users in a targeted discipline, fostering communication and increasing
awareness of both the collection development process and the choices
facing selectors and scholars.

Definition of Collection Assessment

Collection assessment may be defined as the process of measuring or
determining the degree to which a library actually acquired the books,
journals, and other materials it intended to acquire, especially in relation to
the library's collection development policy. "Collection evaluation is concerned with how good a collection is in terms of the kinds of materials in it
and the value of each item in relation to items not in the collection, to the
community being served, and to the library's potential users" [3]. Collection assessment and collection evaluation are terms which are used inter-
changeably in the literature. At the most basic level, collection assessment
or evaluation is a term that encompasses the process of determining the
intrinsic quality of a library's holdings; on a broader level, the term includes
a determination of how well those holdings serve the library's purpose and
meet user information needs [4].

Collection assessment is an integral part of collection development and it provides a systematic measure of the effectiveness of the overall collection development program. At its most fundamental, collection assessment tells how well the selection function is being carried out. Collection assessment has important implications for, and linkages to, a number of other library functions, including reference and public services, interlibrary lending and borrowing, cataloging, acquisitions, and preservation. The data as well as the experience of participation in collection assessment studies can have beneficial applications beyond collection development. The collection development policy should serve as the standard for the collection assessment program.

Reasons for Assessment

Some of the uses for the data from collection assessment studies have been noted previously. The reasons for undertaking such an effort in a library may derive from those uses. In addition to determining the effectiveness of the acquisitions program and its procedures in the implementation of collection development policy and to enhance the service capabilities of the library, other reasons that may motivate collection assessment studies include

- To identify and address weaknesses or gaps in the collections.
- To determine preservation priorities.
- To provide information for collection enhancement.
- To provide information for collection description.
- To allow a library to define or crystallize that which is most central in a local collection and to define priorities for providing access to external resources.
- To enhance the skills of collection development staff by intense exposure to a subject or format.
- To place the library's collection in perspective with the collections of other similar libraries.
- To provide information for cooperative collection development programs.
- To verify a library's collection strengths as reported to regional or national collection inventory projects such as the RLG Conspectus [5] and the North American Collections Inventory Project [6].

- To increase understanding of the literature of various disciplines in the health sciences.

- To redirect and, in some instances, to reduce acquisitions expenditures through the identification and elimination of redundant purchases.

- To determine the ability of the collection to support a new research, clinical, or academic program.

- To participate in accreditation surveys.

- To identify candidates for storage or weeding.

- To gather data for fundraising by identifying areas for endowment and grant support.

- To understand use patterns.

The professional literature of collection evaluation and assessment in research and academic libraries is fairly extensive, including a substantial literature on "weeding." Especially useful sources include Nisonger's *Collection Evaluation in Academic Libraries: a Literature Guide and Annotated Bibliography* [7], Lockett's *Guide to the Evaluation of Library Collections* [8], and Hall's *Collection Assessment Manual for College and University Libraries* [9]. By contrast, the literature on collection assessment in health sciences libraries is relatively sparse, though there is a large literature discussing publication patterns and the development of the literatures of health sciences disciplines. Both of these literatures should be drawn upon as necessary to support a collection assessment program.

Planning Steps

An overall collection assessment program may be viewed as a series of discrete projects governed by a common philosophy and plan. The planning steps for each project may be influenced or dictated by the particular topic, but several steps will be common to them all.

- Determine scope of the assessment and set goals.

- Survey available resources—financial, personnel, and analytic.

- Determine methodology.

- Develop timetable.

- Identify existing policy and other documentation.

- Conduct assessment.

- Analyze findings.
- Develop recommendations and report.
- Implement recommendations.

Project Focuses

The projects comprising a collection assessment program may focus on practically any aspect of the collection. Studies may be conducted on the following:

- Health sciences subjects, both specific and broad.
- Literature formats, such as journals, monographs, audiovisuals, and practice guidelines.
- Collecting levels as stated in the collection development policy.
- Literature types, such as government documents, theses, and annual reports.
- Options for format replacement such as microform sets or runs of periodicals.
- Materials produced to support a particular purpose such as patient education, reference, etc.
- Materials in a selected non-English language or language group.
- Materials published in a selected country or region.
- Materials published during discrete time periods.
- Materials written by or about a particular author or institution.

The implementation of a collection assessment program will be dictated by the local situation, but it is useful for any type and size of library to institute a routine for evaluating the collection subject-by-subject, section-by-section. A small number of major assessment projects may be identified for completion and a schedule drawn up. Additional projects may be scheduled if personnel and other resources become available. Smaller, more discrete projects focused on formats or topics should also be scheduled, especially in connection with other collection development activities.

Methods

There is no single, universal method for conducting collection assessment projects, and the principal sources cited at the end of this chapter recommend a variety of approaches, especially for comprehensive collection assessment efforts. These methods generally fall into two categories: *quantitative*, or numeric, and *qualitative*, or judgmental.

Quantitative studies are principally efforts to measure the percentage of titles from a particular list or bibliography that are held by the library. They may also include the analysis of citations drawn from a selected group of articles, an examination of data derived from interlibrary lending or borrowing activity, or other use studies.

Qualitative studies are characterized by value judgments and they are frequently bibliographic in nature. Examples of this type of study include checking standard or approved lists of items; seeking advice from subject specialists or other experts and applying that advice to quantitative data; and sampling the opinion of users of a segment of a library collection.

To achieve the goals of most collection assessment programs, the principal methodologies tend to be quantitative, which are the most time intensive methods. They provide substantial statistical data, however, and produce a solid base from which interpretation and planning can be accomplished. The types of lists useful for checking vary from discipline to discipline and format to format, but should include such items as "great works in..."; recommended lists from accrediting agencies; "core list of titles in..."; citation studies, especially those in the basic sciences from the Institute for Scientific Information (ISI); and literature analyses in book and periodical form. For studies focused on publications of a given country or in a particular language, national bibliographies and the expertise of dealers can be used. Expert advice can be sought from professional groups and from individuals with expertise and interest in a topic.

Many sources on collection assessment distinguish among and between methodologies by characterizing them as "collection-centered" or "use-centered" measures. Lockett groups commonly employed methods as follows:

Collection-Centered

- Checking lists, catalogs, and bibliographies.
- Expert review of the collection.
- Compilation of comparative use statistics.
- Application of collection standards.

Use-Centered

- Circulation studies.
- In-house use studies.
- Survey of user opinion.
- Shelf availability studies.
- Analysis of ILL statistics.
- Simulated use studies.
- Citation studies.
- Document delivery tests.

Additional common bibliographic based methods include the following:

- Analysis of bibliographies in standard textbooks.
- Comparison of collection against lists of journals included in abstracts and indexes.
- Use of standard lists such as Brandon/Hill.
- Assessment using national or other regional bibliography.
- Comparison of book vendor files in specific subjects for designated time periods.
- Correlation of library holdings with publisher catalogs.

Pros and Cons of Methods

Any method used in collection assessment will have its positive and negative aspects. These have been compiled in Lockett and other sources, to which the reader is referred. The following examples, derived from Lockett, of some common collection-centered and use-centered methods illustrate the range of pros and cons.

Collection-Centered Methods

Checking Lists, Catalogs, and Bibliographies

"The most widely used method of quantitatively evaluating a library's collection is the list-checking method, a process in which the library's holdings are compared with one or more lists of selected titles" [10]. This method involves identification of, selection from, and checking against local holdings, lists of works in subjects, formats and the like which should be in the collection based on collection development policy. Percentages may be developed or analyses undertaken to identify trends.

Advantages

- Lists provide a defined universe against which to measure the collection.

- There is a wide variety of lists available; they may be comprehensive, specialized, general, selected, standard, clinical, research, didactic or educational sources, format types.

- Many lists are backed by authority or the competence of experts, either librarians or subject specialists.

- Lists can be easily manipulated statistically and adapted to the individual library situation.

- List searching does not require special skills or training; existing library staff skills can be utilized; no need for specialized training in statistics or analysis.

- List examination can be a staff development tool; lists can assist in expanding the knowledge of the literature.

- This method may be applied to any type of collection in any type of library.

Disadvantages

- Available lists may have been used as buying guides for the collection under evaluation.

- Lists may not reflect items of interest for the local collection.

- Lists may represent only the viewpoint of one individual and thus not represent the subject in an objective fashion.

- Many standard lists are not revised and may become out of date.

- In some subjects, lists may not be readily available and may require a cumbersome compilation effort.

Expert Review

Expert review may include direct examination of collection, review of "recommended" catalogs, or review of serial lists. It is an inductive process for which the library may engage an outside subject expert or another librarian to conduct a systematic review of the existing collection. This method is most practical with smaller collections, but can be effectively used in larger settings working with segments of a collection or being guided by the user group.

Advantages

- The strengths and weaknesses of the collection can be evaluated relatively rapidly.
- It is easier to achieve multiple objectives such as weeding, identification of items for preservation, replacement, or updating.

Disadvantages

- Specialists may be difficult to locate.
- Specialists may be too expensive for the library budget.
- Specialists may be too busy.
- Results may not be comparable or quantifiable.
- If directly examining a collection physically, some items may be in circulation or not on the shelf, requiring follow-up activities or use of other files.

Use-Centered Methods

Circulation Studies

Collection use studies frequently involve analysis of various types of circulation data, such as direct check-out, in-house use, ILL patterns, and other types of collection use data which may be readily available or which may be gathered specifically for this purpose. This type of study can be used to identify portions of the collection not heavily used, as well as the identification of most heavily used portions of the collection. Collection use studies can also help describe use patterns generally and in specific subjects.

Advantages

- Data are easily arranged into categories for analysis.
- This type of study allows great flexibility as to time frame for study and for sample sizes.
- Units are easily counted.

- Information is objective.
- Correlation with user group segments is easier.

Disadvantages

- It may be difficult to include in-house use so one may not be able to get a complete picture.
- Circulation typically reflects only successes and does not record user or collection failures.
- Data may be biased by inaccessibility of highly used materials, i.e., things may not be available.
- This type of study is generally not useful for collections devoted largely to periodicals, unless the periodical volumes are bar-coded and can be scanned easily.

Survey of User Opinion

The goal of user surveys is to determine how well the collection meets the needs of users. This goal is achieved by gathering oral or written responses to specific questions. User surveys can be controversial and unpredictable, and generally are the hardest to interpret meaningfully. This type of study can however be effective in refining the categories of library users, identifying groups which can be better served, providing feedback, improving public relations, identifying changing trends and interests.

Advantages

- User surveys are extremely flexible and variable and can be simple or complex as required.
- This type of study can be tailored to derive very specialized data, only general data, both specialized and general data, or information about a total user group or segments of the user group.
- These studies can be ongoing or limited to specific time period and can be easily repeated.
- User surveys permit direct feedback from users.

Disadvantages

- Designing a useful survey can be very difficult because it is not easy to frame unambiguous questions that will yield quantifiable results.
- Data analysis is frequently cumbersome, difficult, and imprecise because of open-ended questions.

- Most users are passive about collections and thus must be approached individually and polled one at a time, increasing the time, effort, and ultimately the costs of the survey.

- User cooperation is not always easy to secure.

- Users frequently do not have a realistic expectation or sophisticated awareness of what the library collection should or can contain or understand the collection development policy that guides the selection process.

- User surveys frequently record anecdotal evidence which does not always reflect actual experiences with the collection or true patterns of user behavior.

- User interests may be more narrowly focused than the collection development policy and this may introduce a negative bias in the survey results.

- By definition, user surveys will miss valuable information from and about the nonuser.

Citation Studies

This method can be especially useful in journal dependent collections and for assessments in which the goal is the identification of titles for cancellation or removal. Citation analysis involves counting or ranking citations in published works. There are two basic types:

The first type is published studies such as those that appear in *Current Contents* and other ISI publications; these are based on citation patterns which arise from many scholars in many institutions. The second type is studies that focus on literature in a particular library, especially as that literature supported or did not support work reported in articles by institutional staff. Ask the question: how many of the works cited in Professor Smith's articles on a topic are available in our library?

Advantages

- Data are easily arranged into categories for analysis.
- The method is sufficiently simple that it can be used repeatedly.
- Lists can be compiled efficiently, frequently rapidly, using online databases and other sources.

Disadvantages

- It may be difficult to select source items that truly reflect user group needs and that reflect adequately the subject under scrutiny.
- Subdisciplines may have citation patterns or rates at variance with the overall discipline.
- Time lag for citations may result in a distorted view of the discipline being studied.
- The most cited studies may be inappropriate for the library's collection.

Personnel for Collection Assessments

Staff from all areas of the library should be encouraged to participate in collection assessment studies. Individuals who will assume primary roles in the program are those staff members with selection responsibility. Other staff types who may be called upon include catalogers, reference librarians, format experts, and subject specialists. Technical support staff will generally be expected to complete bibliographic checking tasks, and assistance with statistical interpretation and computational methods may be sought from outside the library. An individual staff member or a group of staff should be identified to conduct an assessment study. Librarians with selection responsibility should include assessment studies as an ongoing part of their responsibilities.

Reports

Written reports with a description of the project, methods employed, data derived, and an analysis of the findings should be done at the conclusion of each project. The report should include, where necessary, a draft of a revised collection development policy statement for the topic. Reports can be formatted according to the following outline.

1. Definition of topic and description of objectives.
2. Statement of scope of project.
3. Documentation, lists.
4. Methodology.
5. Findings
   a. Description of existing collection.

    b. Other collections (as appropriate).
    c. Strengths and weaknesses.
  6. Analysis.
  7. Recommendations and plan for enhancement.
  8. Personnel.

Reports should be shared within the library and with users and outside agencies as appropriate. A centralized and comprehensive file of collection assessment studies should be established and maintained.

Serials Review Projects

Since early in the 1980s, the continued growth in the volume of the health sciences serial literature and the rising costs of that literature have precipitated assessments of serials collections. The approaches to this task have varied, depending on the institution and the urgency with which the projects have been undertaken. The length of time devoted to this type of analysis has a direct relationship to the reliability of the information that results and the use to which that data can be put. Unfortunately the principal motivating factor—subscription cost—too frequently takes precedence over the *need* for the item, and the result is collection development using the "purse-strings" method. Clearly, a more systematic methodology is preferred.

Many smaller libraries review their subscription lists each year and are able to respond to budget pressures in a consistent and rational way. Other health sciences libraries have instituted more stringent practices for library users to follow in recommending new subscriptions, such as expecting justification for the recommendation or requiring a recommendation for cancellation of an existing title before the new subscription can be entered. Larger libraries, in recognition of the continued upward spiral of both new titles and costs, have implemented long-term projects that allow the library to rationalize the selection decisions through prioritization and consideration of additional factors to subscription cost. They are then able to accommodate budget concerns more easily and can preserve the integrity of the primary part of the collection. The elements of this type of assessment activity parallel those already described for other evaluation projects.

A recent survey [11] on serials review projects in academic health sciences libraries revealed that more than half indicated that a systematic review of the library's entire serials collection had been undertaken. Of the libraries at which a systematic review of the entire collection had been done, more than half provided brief descriptions of the process or of the criteria that were considered. The reviews were usually subject-based, that is, the library's journal list was divided into broad subjects and lists of titles in the subject were prepared. These lists were then reviewed by the primary users in that discipline or by all library users. The most commonly used alternative to subject listings was a list of titles arranged by subscription price.

All processes involved library users to some degree, either through memoranda to faculty and departments, through notices in library newsletters, or through special meetings involving library staff and user groups. Several institutions relied on existing serials review committees to conduct the review, whereas others concentrated the responsibility in a specially appointed group or in collection development staff.

Most institutions indicated that library staff and library users shared the decision-making process, though several libraries firmly stated that the library staff retained the decision-making power and that user input was advisory only. In several institutions, users were asked to assign priorities to titles on lists of potential cancellations that had been identified by library staff. These rankings were then used to identify a targeted dollar amount.

The most commonly cited criteria that were considered were use and cost, with the latter more often driving the process. Frequently, consideration was given to institutional duplication of the title, especially when the review process involved academic medical libraries that are parts of university library systems. ILL statistics, whether the journal was indexed in major abstracting tools, and *Science Citation Index* "impact factor" were other criteria that figured prominently in some review processes. Programmatic relevance, that is, the degree to which the title is related to academic, research, or clinical programs, appeared in only a few instances, perhaps because the "fat" had long since been trimmed from serials lists and the processes being used currently are based on an assumption that only relevant titles are being acquired.

A recommended methodology for libraries to consider is outlined in Table 9-1. The intention here is to present a range of options under each category, not to prescribe or to suggest that every library need undertake all steps. The plan can be adapted for any type of library by the omission or addition of specific local concerns.

Collection Assessments for a New Institutional Program

A particular type of collection assessment exercise is required when a new educational program, research effort, or clinical enterprise must be factored into an existing collection development program. The following steps and guidelines can be useful both in determining what new support

Table 9-1: Generic Serials Review Project Plan

I. Statement of Project Goals:

A. To review the current subscription list in light of recently revised collection development guidelines and to remove titles that no longer meet the guidelines, and to add, if possible, titles that are missing.
B. To articulate to segments of the library's user group (departments, faculty, institutes, etc.), the library's collection development policy for appropriate disciplines, and to refine that policy based on user input.
C. To heighten user awareness of the selection process and of the costs and numbers of health science related "new" publications.
D. To enhance and encourage library user involvement in the selection process for serials.
E. To identify emerging needs, especially of new programs and rapidly expanding fields.

II. Project Guidelines

A. The project is conducted by the library's serials selection committee, and is incorporated into the routine work of the committee.
B. The project is a subject-based review wherein all current subscriptions in a given subject are reviewed together.
C. The project requires review both by library staff and by library users in affected departments and institutes.
D. A variety of factors is considered in determining whether to continue or to discontinue a title, or whether to add a title not currently held; these factors include the following.

1. Bibliographic accessibility of the title in major abstracting and indexing services.
2. The availability of the title at other institutional libraries or through network agreements.
3. The continued relevance of the title to the actual or potential needs of research, clinical, or educational programs of the user group.
4. Scope and content of the title.
5. Quality.
6. Price.
7. Language and country of origin.
8. Type of publication.
9. Use of the title insofar as it can be determined (interlibrary lending data; circulation figures: in-house use).
10. Regional commitments to retain titles under cooperative collection development arrangements.
11. The level of coverage of the subject as reflected in the Research Libraries Group Conspectus or other comparative library measures.

E. Additionally, an effort should be made to define a universe of titles for the subject beyond those held by the library conducting the serials review. Intellectual satisfaction would dictate that the full universe of titles within a given subject be identified; practical considerations, however, mitigate against that level of activity. Subject lists may be identified and checked as part of a subject review but comprehensive efforts are generally impractical. User input on policy and on additional titles should be sought.

F. A timetable for the project should be established and periodic reports prepared.

III. Methodology

A. The library's serials selection committee, with input from the library advisory committee and other sources, identifies priorities and categories of subscriptions which it is not necessary to review, e.g., titles indexed in *Abridged Index Medicus*, classic or standard titles in the discipline.
B. The library's current serials list should be divided into approximately fifty subject categories reflecting RLG conspectus categories or some other systematic subject division.
C. A serials review project form should be designed and completed for each title, including title-specific information as reflected above.
D. The serials selection committee should examine sample issues or volumes for each title and make a preliminary decision to continue or discontinue each title.
E. The list of titles within the subject should be compiled and circulated for comment by the faculty and other users in the departments that may be users of the titles; at the same time, users should be asked to identify titles not currently held that should be considered by the serials selection committee.
F. User input should be incorporated into a final retention or cancellation decision to be made for each title within the group.
G. The library should implement the decisions as the review of each subject file is completed and should revise as necessary the collection development policy statement for the subject.
H. A summary report of the individual subject review should be compiled and distributed to the department and within the library system.
I. At the conclusion of the project, a summary of all actions should be prepared and distributed.

---

is required and how the existing collection meets the needs of the new program.

Understand the Program

1. Identify the disciplines that are related to or relevant for the new program and determine the level of collection that already exists. Do not assume that you will need to purchase large amounts of new material to support the new program. The literature of the health sciences is highly interrelated, e.g., the literature of AIDS derives from immunology, public health, epidemiology, infectious diseases, sexually transmitted diseases, basic physiology; the literature of biotechnology from biochemistry, genetics, molecular biology, structural biochemistry.
2. Obtain a copy of the statement of purpose for the new program. Analyze that document to determine such things as the following: the precise nature of the research (laboratory or literature based?); the range of courses to be taught; the type and level of care to be

provided; the number of individuals involved; the length, source and level of funding.

3. Identify the key researchers, educators, and practitioners and their specific interests. Meet with them to discuss library support and request copies of relevant documents, such as research proposals, course syllabi, which would provide information that can be used to define the scope of the new program. Also determine their plans for meeting their own information needs and those of their colleagues. Codify to the degree possible those information needs.

4. Talk with the institutional grants office or related organizational entity to get on the mailing list for information about future grants or proposals submitted and approved.

Understand the Literature of the Field

1. Identify key current and retrospective bibliographies, textbooks, recommended lists, and journals in the subject. Conduct systematic checking of these sources against the existing collection. Track established use patterns to ascertain the need for additional copies of works already in the collection.

2. Review a few introductory works or articles to get a feel for the field.

3. To determine the degree of ongoing budget support required, calculate the publishing output, e.g., new books published per year for the discipline, and current serial titles. Especially helpful for this exercise are analyses of approval plan programs from major booksellers and subject analyses of health sciences serials done by serials agents.

Identify Other Available Resources

1. Identify other collections that have been developed to support similar programs in other places. Contact librarians in those institutions to discuss their experiences in developing responsive collections and assessing existing ones, and the possibilities for cooperative collection development.

2. Determine which resources should be in the local collection and which can be stored if accessible. Define priorities for local and remote access in light of print resources.

Using the information derived from the above steps, (1) develop new collection development policies or adjust existing ones to accommodate the new program; (2) develop budget projections and statements of justification for whatever augmentation to the materials budgets is required; and (3) identify other effects of the new program on existing library services such as educational programs, reference, course reserves, cataloging.

References

1. Mosher PH. Collection evaluation or analysis: matching library acquisitions to library needs. In Stueart RD, Miller GB, eds. Collection development in libraries: a treatise, pt.B. Greenwich, CT: JAI Press, 1980:6.

2. Metcalf KD. The National Library of Medicine; report of a survey of the Army Medical Library. Chicago: American Library Association, 1944.

3. Magrill RM, Corbin J. Acquisition management and collection development in libraries. 2d ed. Chicago: American Library Association, 1989:234.

4. Nisonger TE. Collection evaluation in academic libraries: a literature guide and annotated bibliography. Englewood, CO: Libraries Unlimited, 1992:ix.

5. Ferguson AW, Grant J, Rutstein JS. The RLG conspectus: its uses and benefits. Coll Res Libr 1988 May;49(3):197-206.

6. Branin J, Farrell D, Tiblin M. The National Shelflist Count Project: its history, limitations, and usefulness. Libr Res Tech Serv 1985 Oct/Dec;29(4):333-342.

7. Nisonger, op. cit.

8. Lockett, B, ed. Guide to the evaluation of library collections. Chicago: American Library Association, 1989. (Collection management and development guides, no. 2).

9. Hall BH. Collection assessment manual for college and university libraries. Phoenix, AZ: Oryx Press, 1985.

10. Comer CH. List-checking as a method of evaluating library collections. In Sellen BC, Curley A, eds. The collection building reader. New York : Neal-Schuman, 1992:174.

11. Richards DT, Prelec A. Serials cancellation projects: necessary evil or collection assessment opportunity? J Libr Admin 1992; 17(2):31-45.

10

Cooperative Collection Development

"Cooperation is not an activity libraries may or may not choose to engage in—it is the element in which they live and prosper. Cooperation is an essential to a library as is water to a fish or air to a mammal."

Michael Gorman, 1986

The introduction to *Standards for Cooperative Multitype Library Organizations* opens with the following lines:

> Cooperation among libraries is not a new phenomenon and, indeed, over a century of cooperation among librarians in the United States makes up the heritage of present day practitioners. That libraries should be able to work cooperatively to find access to information in distant collections which is not available locally is a deeply rooted concept in librarianship [1].

Cooperation is fundamental to the operation of libraries and, among and between libraries, has taken many forms. Partnerships large and small participate in interlibrary lending and borrowing, purchase materials collectively, offer reciprocal access privileges to users, develop storage facilities, manage joint technical processing systems, and provide reference services. Each of these can be called resource sharing in its broadest definition. The focus of this chapter is the library collection itself and how cooperation among and between institutions can play an important role in meeting the information needs of a library's users. (For further information on library cooperation refer to Volume 7 in this series, *Health Sciences Environment and Librarianship in Health Sciences Libraries*.)

Definition

Cooperative collection development occurs when two or more libraries coordinate their collection building activities in some agreed upon way. It should be seen as a "subset of activities in the larger realm of library cooperation" [2]. Branin has defined three cooperative activities that comprise the subset: mutual notification of purchasing decisions; joint purchase; and assigned subject specialization in acquisitions [3]. Mosher and Pankake authored the first set of recommended guidelines for designing and implementing cooperative collection development ventures among libraries [4]. According to this guide, cooperative collection development involves the sharing of responsibilities among two or more libraries for the purpose of acquiring materials, developing collections, and managing the growth and maintenance of collections in a user- beneficial and cost-beneficial way [5].

A newer publication from ALA brings the earlier work up to date but reiterates many of the same principles [6]. It also discusses the benefits of cooperative collection development, provides definitions of terms, identifies pitfalls of cooperative collection development, and serves as a useful guide to librarians and administrators wishing to initiate cooperative collection development programs. The rationales for cooperative collection development, as well as the potential problems, issues, models, and policies are not significantly different for health sciences libraries from those which affect other kinds of libraries. Consequently, this guide is a very useful tool for health sciences librarians contemplating cooperative collection development.

Goals

Cooperative collection development programs and arrangements frequently grow out of a desire to use existing materials budgets more effectively. The goal may be to reduce unnecessary overlap or duplication between collections while maintaining or expanding the universe of materials available in the combined collections of the participants. Another motive might be to ensure that materials currently available to users in a given geographic area are not lost inadvertently through uncoordinated collection development decisions. Still other reasons for cooperating include

- The coordination of cancellations, storage, or preservation decisions in comparable collections.

- An enhanced understanding of the collection development processes in other types of libraries and coordination of planning for collection development.

- The establishment among larger research collections of library of record status or primary collection responsibilities for specific subjects and formats.

- The acquisition of collective site licenses for databases of common interest among user groups.

- Distribution among smaller closely neighboring libraries of certain core or basic subjects in order to reduce unwanted or insupportable redundancy.

These potential reasons for entering into cooperative agreements can also be viewed as potential benefits to be gained from such arrangements.

Cooperative collection development, or resource building, assumes a commitment to resource sharing as well. Resource sharing is commonly defined as the sharing of library collections through one or more of the following mechanisms:

- The provision of information on what cooperating institutions own.
- The actual interlibrary lending and borrowing of materials.
- Direct service to the user populations of cooperating libraries.

Resource sharing, however, is not "...simply a matter of improved bibliographic access, or better document delivery, or more cooperative collection development, but a combination of activities in all three areas..." [7]. Irrespective of the scope of the resource sharing program, cooperative collection development is meaningless without both a commitment among participating institutions to share their collections and an effective mechanism to do so.

Cooperative Collection Development in the Health Sciences

The history of resource sharing is a long and distinguished one, especially among health sciences libraries. Productive resource-sharing arrangements among health sciences librarians began with the creation of the MLA Exchange in the late nineteenth century. Cooperative collection development, as distinct from resource sharing, however, is a relatively recent phenomenon, though it may properly be regarded as a refinement, inevitable or not, of resource sharing. Although the majority of activity in cooperative collection development has been among large research libraries, there have been some cooperative programs in other types of libraries as well. While there are many examples of cooperative collection development programs that have been devised and operated for discrete periods of time, there are few programs in existence today.

Cooperative collection development programs did arise in the formerly named Regional Medical Library (RML) network. Indeed, all of the activities under the general rubric "cooperation" are found in abundance in the RML and described by Bunting [8]. Resource-sharing programs in the RML specifically were designed "to share information resources and coordinate the development of regional collections" [9]. Some ensure retention of important serial titles within a specific region; others expand the monographs available among health sciences libraries. These programs tend to include libraries of varying types and sizes.

Examples of past cooperative collection development programs in health sciences libraries include the serials rationalization program and the Cooperative Acquisitions Program (CAP) of the South Central Regional Medical Library Program, formerly called TALON. Under the serials program, libraries participating in a union list agreed to continue subscriptions to a core set of titles [10]. The program also included the regular distribution of "add" and "drop" lists to partners, and the shifting of back files from library to library to complete sets. CAP was predicated on the notion that participating libraries assumed responsibility for acquiring books from selected publishers within a profile covering subject and format [11]. These programs were moderately successful but, ironically, were discontinued in the face of budget pressures [12].

The Cooperative Serials Acquisitions Program (COSAP) of the Pacific Southwest Regional Medical Library Service (PSRMLS) is another example of an RML-sponsored effort. The resource libraries in PSRMLS agreed to continue subscriptions to journals held by fewer than three libraries [13]. The focus of the program was on the esoteric and costs for subscriptions maintained by participating University of California (UC) libraries were funded by the University's shared acquisitions program. The program was discontinued due to budgetary pressures and the redirection of UC shared acquisitions program funds to database licensing costs for the MELVYL system.

Another example of a cooperative serials retention program is the Regional Coordination of Biomedical Information Resources Program, commonly called RECBIR [14]. The primary purpose of RECBIR, which began as an activity of the Medical Library Center of New York (MLCNY) but which in 1983 became an RML program, is to ensure local availability of health sciences periodicals for a large geographic region and to provide cooperative insurance that those titles will not be lost through indiscriminate cancellation. It is not a cooperative acquisitions program, because no funds change hands, but rather a cooperative retention program. This is accomplished through a program of voluntary commitments on the part of several hundred libraries to maintain subscriptions to titles indexed in *List of Serials Indexed for Online Users*. RECBIR has undergone a number of adjustments over time but it continues today. No formal evaluation of its effectiveness has been undertaken.

The development of audiovisual collections and media centers in health sciences libraries spurred the sharing of audiovisual materials through traditional interlibrary borrowing and lending activities. Cooperative purchase arrangements have also occurred, though only on a modest level. A 1987 survey of 132 United States and Canadian medical school libraries documented that thirty-one libraries at that time participated in some form of audiovisual resource sharing [15]. Of those, sixteen indicated that they were involved in cooperative collection development.

Even though the number of existing cooperative collection development arrangements among health sciences libraries is not particularly high, the administrative and bibliographic structures they have developed to support interlibrary loan and exchange of duplicates provide an excellent basis for further work in this area. These structures provide health science librarians with a solid base upon which to build and refine more comprehensive collection development agreements.

Difficulties

"Cooperative collection development is at its most basic level a political, not a technical, issue" [16]. Whatever form that activity takes, the management of the activity transcends local autonomous boundaries. Cooperative collection development is not regarded with pleasure in all circles. Agreements to develop collections in a coordinated way may run afoul of local priorities and operations in individual libraries. "Library planning and collection building in research libraries of the United States have long had to deal with two contradictory forces, autonomy and independence" [17]. This same observation can be made for health sciences libraries and is something that any library contemplating cooperative collection development must face.

Other difficulties that have presented themselves include institutional rivalries, particularly between and among faculties at different institutions. These have arisen when libraries in those institutions have developed cooperative collection development programs. Financial exigencies too have created problems for libraries in cooperative agreements, which, regardless of arrangements made with great good will in more prosperous times, can no longer be honored. Last, a subject-based arrangement for cooperative collection development may be difficult to sustain if at a later time the importance of the subject to the institution diminishes because of a change in institutional philosophy or educational focus.

Requirements

The underlying reason for all cooperative collection development and library resource sharing is the knowledge that no single library can contain all the information its users need or want. While resource sharing can be viewed as providing access to what other libraries have acquired, cooperative collection development is an active attempt to influence what is acquired and therefore expand the universe of material available to be shared. If a library wishes to explore cooperative programs, there is no single model for such arrangements. There are some basic requirements, beginning with the design and support of an effective organization for cooperation, an organizational entity that has the political ability to negotiate inevitable conflicts of interest and the power to administer complex programs over distance and time [18].

Cooperative agreements can be developed among libraries within a single institution, among libraries of a single type, of different types, or along regional or geographic lines. Frequently, cooperative collective agreements arise among institutions that already have some other form of cooperative mechanism established. The range of possible collection development arrangements is enormous, but the requirements of the participants should include

- A clear concept of the missions of the institutions the libraries serve and the way the libraries support their missions.

- An understanding of the present and future information needs of the user groups of the libraries.
- A knowledge of the existing strengths and weaknesses of the library collections.
- An accurate picture of current collecting practices.
- Use data for the library collections, important because these data are evidence of the present user demands on a local collection, demands which should not be compromised by new demands from the user groups of partner libraries.

With the exception of the last of these requirements, all should be present in a well-drafted collection development policy statement. Once these requirements have been satisfied, the library must decide if it has a reasonable basis for cooperative action in collection development. The probability of profitable cooperative collection development is more limited if the requirements of the participating institutions are largely overlapping and each institution acquires only core materials. A viable agreement must be a "win-win" proposition, and each participant must feel the agreement supports the individual library's goals and serves the needs of the user group.

The parameters of an agreement must take into account a wide variety of concerns beyond the selection process, including processing, retention, use, fees, and preservation. Procedures established should involve a minimum of additional work for participants and should provide a method for gathering statistics and costs for future evaluation. All of these factors should be reduced to a written agreement, much like a contract, which is signed by all parties. The overall goal of any cooperative effort should be to minimize unnecessary duplication and to broaden the available resources. The success of the effort will turn on access to the material acquired under the agreement.

The Future

Cooperative collection development programs during the last century have risen and fallen largely because of the effectiveness or carelessness of consortial arrangements. Local...programs have fared relatively well because administering such programs is a much simpler matter [19].

The future for cooperation in resource building and sharing among health sciences libraries appears to be bright. That brightness though is diminished by the aggressive efforts of groups such as the Association of American Publishers (AAP) to impose more stringent requirements on cooperative collection development. A recent AAP position paper on document delivery attempts to cast resource sharing of copies provided under interlibrary lending and borrowing as "systematic" copying [20]. Though the document does not address shared purchasing or cooperative collection development specifically, it is indicative of a trend which must be considered.

Many of the factors that prescribe cooperation will only increase, as there seems to be no drop in the volume of materials being added to the information base. There is also significant potential for cooperative collection development among libraries with rare, unique, and valuable resources; programs in this type of library can be effectively structured to build on existing strengths of the collections. As libraries articulate, in a more systematic way, their policies and practices regarding collection development, the opportunities for cooperative resource building will increase. Further, as health sciences libraries find it more difficult to afford secondary and tertiary materials needed by their users, the benefits of expanding cooperative agreements with other libraries will become even more compelling.

Electronic networks and linkages can enhance significantly the delivery of information, and, by doing so, expand the range of information resources available to a library's user group. Harloe and Budd state that "In a networked environment, it is possible for academic libraries to move beyond the rhetoric of 'access versus ownership' " to the development of a collection that is in fact a network of connections rather than a local or cooperative physical collection [21].

Such a shift has long-range implications for cooperative collection development, among which is instilling in the mind of the local user the view of the library as a gateway rather than a repository. The potential for this alone may require a rethinking of the cooperative collection development paradigm if not library cooperation in its broadest sense. Bunting noted that the greatest challenge to the RML program is to facilitate the development of an electronic system so that pertinent information from all types of repositories can be accessed using a common communications protocol [22]. As Sheila Dowd eloquently observed:

> Information is the raw stuff from which knowledge is derived; but information must be organized to foster connections and relevant interpretations before it will lead to knowledge. Life is not a trivia game. Bits and bytes of information are important only if the mind can link them with other pieces of information to build the orderly patterns that are the fabric of knowledge. Hence the mission of

libraries is more properly identified as the provision of access to organized information, for the fostering of knowledge [23].

The challenge to health sciences librarians is to marshal their considerable collective experience with cooperative programs to provide mechanisms for improved access to health sciences information. National, regional and local cooperative collection development programs have the potential both to improve information service to health professionals and to permit more effective use of increasingly limited library resources. These potential benefits are real and deserve careful consideration in all health sciences library collection development efforts.

References

1. Association of Specialized and Cooperative Library Agencies. Standards for cooperative multitype library organizations. Chicago: American Library Association, 1990:1.

2. Branin JJ. Cooperative collection development. In: Osburn CB, Atkinson RW, eds. Collection management: a new treatise. Greenwich, CT: JAI Press, 1991:81. (Foundations in library and information science; v. 26A).

3. Ibid., 81.

4. Mosher PH, Pankake M. A guide to coordinated and cooperative collection development. Libr Res Tech Serv 1983 Oct/Dec;27(4):417-31.

5. Ibid., 419-20.

6. Harloe B, ed. Guide to cooperative collection development. Chicago: American Library Association, 1994. (ALCTS Collection management and development guides, no. 6.)

7. Branin, op. cit., 82.

8. Bunting A. The nation's health information network: history of the Regional Medical Library Program, 1965-85. Bull Med Libr Assoc 1987 Jul;75(3, supp.):1-62.

9. Ibid., 27.

10. Hendricks DD. TALON—the first five years. Bull Med Libr Assoc 1976 Apr;64(2):206-7.

11. Kronick DA. A regional cooperative acquisitions program for monographs. Bull Med Libr Assoc 1979 Jul;67(3):297-300.

12. Bowden VM, Comeaux EA, Eakin D. Evaluation of TALON Cooperative Acquisitions Program for monographs. Bull Med Libr Assoc 1984 Jul;72(3):241-50.

13. Bunting A. Region XI Cooperative Serials Acquisitions Project (COSAP). Terminal progress report. Los Angeles: Biomedical Library, PSRMLS, January 1, 1979.

14. Jones CL. A cooperative serial acquisition program: thoughts on a response to mounting fiscal pressures. Bull Med Libr Assoc 1974 Apr;62(2):120-3.

15. Richards DT, Curtis JA. Audiovisual resource sharing in medical school libraries: a status report. Unpublished presentation at the 88th Annual Meeting of the Medical Library Association, New Orleans, LA, May 22, 1988.

16. Branin, op. cit., 104-5.

17. Stam DH. Collaborative collection development: progress, problems, and potential. In: Sellen BC, Curley A, eds. The collection building reader. New York: Neal-Schuman, 1992:201.

18. Branin, op. cit., 105.

19. Ibid.

20. Association of American Publishers. Statement of the Association of American Publishers (AAP) on commercial and fee-based document delivery. Washington, DC: Association of American Publishers, 1992.

21. Harloe B, Budd JM. Collection development and scholarly communication in the era of electronic access. J Acad Libr 1994 May;20(2):83-7.

22. Bunting A. The nation's health information network, op. cit., 48.

23. Dowd ST. Library cooperation: methods, models to aid information access. J Libr Admin 1990;12(3):63-81.

11

Preservation

"Child! Do not throw this book about;
Refrain from the untold pleasure
of cutting all the pictures out!
Preserve it as your chiefest treasure."

Hilaire Belloc, 1896

Health sciences libraries exist as both information centers and repositories of the published and unpublished records of the health sciences. The collection of materials to support the information center function of the library is ever changing, and must be timely, of high quality, and responsive to the information needs of the library's constituent user groups. A library's collection development program draws from the large and ever-growing output of the publishing industry. For this reason, the selection process must be based on a mechanism that assists in the making of choices; it is only at the level of a "special" collection that any library can aspire to assemble a collection that includes all materials its users might potentially require. Most cooperative efforts among libraries are based on a recognition of that fact. Consequently, the notion that a single institution can be self-sufficient is rarely in evidence among medical libraries today.

An effective collection development program provides the framework within which to make choices. Selection criteria form an integral part of that framework. These criteria are weighed with or against each other in the decision process and can assume greater or lesser importance from item to item. With few exceptions, they may be effectively applied in the preservation process, because selection for preservation is, in effect, a "reselection" decision.

Selection for preservation in the health sciences requires, as well, an awareness of the literature of the health sciences, in particular the scholarly record and its components. Despite the imprecision in the number of items in the scholarly record of biomedicine, the numbers are significant, and all of these collections combined result in a scholarly record for biomedicine that comprises many millions of items. To preserve them all is likely unnecessary and may well be beyond the capabilities and economics of modern technology. As Oliver Wendell Holmes observed in his *Medical Essays:*

> Our shelves contain many books which only a certain class of medical scholars will be likely to consult. There is a dead medical literature, and there is a live one. The dead is not all ancient, the live is not all modern. There is none, modern or ancient, which, if it has no living value for the student, will not teach him something by its autopsy [1].

Selection for Preservation in Other Disciplines

As stated by Philip H. Abelson in *Science*, one of the "Stimuli for scholarly publication is the belief by scientists and other authors that their work will add enduring values to the human heritage" [2]. The deteriorating condition of millions of books and journals belies that hope, and preservation inventories conducted in many major libraries make clear the extent of the problem. More than a quarter of the holdings of the Library of Congress, some three million volumes, are already too brittle to handle and an additional 77,000 volumes become brittle annually. The National Library of Medicine book and journal collection numbers in excess of 2,000,000. Of that number, preservation surveys indicate that some 12.8% is embrittled and in need of preservation microfilming. It is not unusual for preservation inventories to report that 35-40% of a library collection requires preservation attention. Preservation of materials is an immediate and essential issue for all libraries.

There is a wealth of information and a wide spectrum of publications focused on preservation issues: the extent of the problem, the methods available for restoration or replacement, and the financial resources needed. Clark edited a very useful guide for the selection of materials that should be preserved [3]. This publication provides in a concise format a review of the literature, individual library policies, definitions of terms, discussion of methodologies for collection surveys, and an extensive bibliography on the topic. Slote's valuable guide [4] to the weeding process can have utility in most selection for preservation routines.

The selection for preservation process follows the basic structure of other selection processes and can be described by asking two fundamental questions: who should make the decisions, and, on what basis should the decisions be made? While there is relative agreement in the profession about the answers to those questions for routine library selection, a literature review finds a variety of approaches, many of which are germane to selection for preservation in the health sciences.

Hazen presents a conceptual framework for individual preservation decisions, stressing that the same considerations for building collections apply to preservation [5]. He offers five factors for consideration as guidelines for preservation selection: 1) academic activity, or user demand; 2) historical precedent and tradition; 3) the volume and cost of materials; 4) the availability of alternatives to purchasing replacements; and 5) discipline-specific access to information. He describes these five factors, first in relation to collection development and then in terms of what should be preserved. He points out the considerable staff time that selection for preservation requires and concludes with a plea that libraries must have better information about the cost and cost-effectiveness of specific preservation options and that it is essential to systematize the existing welter of information on material already available in other formats.

Walker discusses the full spectrum of preservation issues [6]. Pertinent to selection for preservation is the recommendation that there be a staff member to coordinate the process of gathering information about the volumes given to the subject specialist for decisions. The subject bibliographer then determines the fate of each work—whether to restore, repair, withdraw, box, transfer, or replace. If it must be replaced, then further decisions are needed—whether to purchase an available reprint or microform or to photocopy or microfilm, either through commercial services or an in-house program. Walker includes an extensive outline of how to search for the information needed to make informed selection for preservation decisions. These recommendations assume that the library has the staff to carry out systematic searching and decision making. Unfortunately, the recent preservation needs assessment survey of the nation's health sciences libraries, a survey conducted under NLM's Regional Medical Library Program and discussed in detail by Kirkpatrick, reveals that few health sciences libraries have preservation officers or staff dedicated to preservation activities [7].

Atkinson proposes a decision cycle model for selecting for preservation and discusses the technical (what needs preservation and which modes are possible?) and critical (what should be preserved and which mode should be used?) aspects of the model [8]. His response to the fundamental question for preservation—why should certain items survive and others not?—is a second model identified as a typology of preservation, showing three classes of preservation distinguished by four factors. The four factors include the object, that is, the item or collection; the primary mode of preservation; where in the organization decision is made; and the decision type.

In Atkinson's model, **Class 1** preservation includes those resources which will be preserved as artifacts because of their economic value, such as rare books and manuscripts. Also included here are level 5 collections, as defined by the Research Libraries Group (RLG) Conspectus. Such a collection is defined as ". . . one in which the library endeavors, insofar as possible, to include all significant works of recorded knowledge (publications, manuscripts, other forms) in all applicable languages for a necessarily defined and limited field. This level of collecting intensity is one that maintains a 'special collection' the aim, if not the achievement, is exhaustiveness" [9]. These collections may also have significant capital value which derives from the combination of materials or the comprehensiveness of the collection. Preservation decision making is generally of the macro variety and is done at the local level.

Class 2 preservation is represented by heavily used materials in current demand for curricular or research purposes. It is temporal and may be described as conservation. These materials are generally identified as they are returned from circulation. It is here, Atkinson says, that bibliographers have their most important role, using the same criteria they have developed in building the collection to make determinations for preserving it. This category also emphasizes the item-by-item selection called for by Hazen.

Class 3 preservation is more difficult to define, and it is in this area that decisions are made to preserve lower-use research materials for posterity. Development of criteria for preservation selection here is critical, as is cooperation in preservation activities. Atkinson suggests that quantity has become quality in today's research library, principally because of our inability to measure bibliographical quality in any other terms. Because of this, he argues against trying to assign values to items and proposes a coordinated cooperative program for Class 3 materials to insure the preservation of a "representative" collection based on the most distinguished collection in a given discipline.

Child, while generally supporting Atkinson's three classes of preservation, takes issue with his inclusion of level 5 collections in Class 1, and proposes that such ". . . collections must be included within the overall priorities of a cooperative national preservation program. [10]" She also suggests that the dilemma of decision making in Class 3 is more complex than Atkinson described and offers two reasons—the expansion of American research since World War II, which broadened the range of documentation useful for historical research, and the fact that today it is technologically possible to save everything. Child's article focuses on the need for cooperative filming projects that would use the strongest subject collections as their base, but stresses the need to include in the preservation effort other collections as well to insure that the representative collection advocated by Atkinson is achieved.

Bagnall and Harris discuss the importance of involving scholars in the process of selection for preservation, and list two levels for decision making: microdecisions, or, title-by-title choices, and macrodecisions, or, decision at the collection level [11]. They suggest four approaches to preservation selection: 1) the vacuum cleaner approach, where preservation decisions are made for a particular range of dates, or places of publication, within a collection or a subject; 2) the condition-driven approach, where materials are queued for preservation decisions when they can no longer circulate or be used because of their deteriorated condition; 3) the bibliographic model, in which all materials included in a particular bibliography are selected for preservation review and treatment; and, 4) the collection development model, where title-by-title preservation decisions are made by bibliographers and other collection development specialists. These authors advocate a shared responsibility between scholars and librarians for making selection for preservation decisions.

Selection for Preservation in Health Sciences Library Collections

The literature addressing selection for preservation in health sciences libraries is relatively small, consisting principally of articles that have appeared in the *Bulletin of the Medical Library Association,* the most important of which appeared as a symposium in 1989 [12]. The symposium addressed the issue from a variety of perspectives beginning with DeBakey and DeBakey's provocative challenge:

> Scholars, scientists, physicians, other health professionals, and librarians face a crucial decision today: shall we nourish the biomedical archives as a viable and indispensable source of information, or shall we bury their ashes and lose a century or more of consequential scientific history? [13]

They make a compelling case for the need to preserve the biomedical literature for ". . . intellectual, historical, social, cultural, political, and economic reasons. . ." [14].

Byrnes describes the efforts of NLM to preserve the biomedical literature and covers the development of the National Preservation Plan [15]. She exhorts librarians in libraries of all types and sizes to participate in the preservation effort by incorporating preservation practices into daily operations and developing disaster plans among other activities [16]. Kirkpatrick reports the results of a national survey of preservation activities in health sciences libraries. Among his findings from the 231 survey respondents are that basic health sciences libraries are engaged in preservation activities at a minimal level, except for binding. Resource libraries, on the other hand, have addressed the problem more vigorously through the development of preservation plans and designation of staff to implement the plans. He observed that "Most preservation efforts in health sciences libraries . . . were local in scope and were focused on extending the useful lifespan of particular items" [17]. Richards and McClure address selection for preservation [18]. Paulson provided a sample preservation policy and procedures document stressing the importance of raising preservation awareness among library staff and users, as well as setting priorities for preservation within the local collection [19].

A series of articles on weeding health sciences library collections appeared as a *Bulletin of the Medical Library Association* symposium in 1952. The symposium provides some viewpoints which are both interesting and relevant to selection for preservation, because weeding constitutes a decision not to preserve.

The symposium contained five short papers discussing weeding in various types of medical libraries and of various kinds of library materials. The authors advise "caution" as the guiding principle in any weeding effort. Carr states: "First, be absolutely convinced of the necessity of the measure; second, make your selection with the greatest care; and third, dispose of the material so cautiously and surreptitiously that there will be no corpus delicti" [20]. Murphy recommends keeping one copy of each edition of important texts, such as Osler's *Practice of Medicine* and Holt's *Textbook of Pediatrics* because they form "records of the development of these fields" [21]. Felter [22] and Reilley [23] point out the variations in weeding practices in the special hospital library and the association library. The series concludes with advice from Marshall [24] on weeding pamphlet collections.

Duffield proposes a useful list of questions the librarian must answer in considering whether to discard multivolume series, often called cyclopedias, or systems of surgery or medicine [25]. Her eight questions are worth repeating because they are similar to the ones asked today to determine whether or not to retain a title:

1. Does this set contain historical material not found elsewhere in the library?

2. Does this set have historical value as far as your own institution is concerned? Was it edited by a member, or does it contain members' papers not found elsewhere?
3. If you disposed of this set, could you borrow it from a nearby library? What is the expense involved?
4. To your knowledge has this set been referred to in the past five years?
5. Are you serving a state-wide area? Do you feel your library should have everything, regardless of present usage? Why?
6. Do you have housing for little-used or never-used material?
7. Do you intend to dispose of this material as the collection grows and you are faced with the problem of insufficient space?
8. If you have storage for sets that are seldom used, can you get them within an hour? [26]

Several authors, including Meckel [27] relied on Garrison and Morton's *Medical Bibliography* as the first checkpoint in selection for weeding. Any item listed therein should be kept by the library. Duplicate copies of both textbooks and journals, loose-leaf compilations, and reprints were cited as the most likely candidates for withdrawal, although Meckel doubted the need to keep all editions of a textbook.

Patterson calls for more "decisive and courageous" action, declaring that libraries must weed to survive and pointing out that there are depository libraries that can be relied upon [28]. Cooperation in weeding collections can be useful and the Mid-West Regional Centre, now known as the Center for Research Libraries, is cited as an example. Both Meckel and Patterson emphasize the need to establish policies for both acquiring and withdrawing. Finally, Doe in a 1953 editorial called for an ongoing compilation of outstanding publications in medicine, similar to the *Standard Catalog for Public Libraries* [29]. She chides medical librarians for failing to make judgments on the worth of individual items. What a boon such a list would be today in making selection for preservation decisions.

Criteria for Selection for Preservation

Objective scholarly testimony in the form of a recommendation on a list or through other means is important in determining whether to preserve an individual item. Of equal importance is the retention and preservation of a collection that represents not just the best in a subject, but the typical; not just the current, but the widest range of years. Librarians once collected to meet the needs of current library users but also collected for the future user. This role for most libraries today is significantly diminished because of the primary role NLM has taken in this arena. The largest medical library collections contain important unique materials and should, of course, preserve them. DeBakey says

> Our vast pre-electronic archives also help us understand the nature and progression of research—the ambiguities, false starts, contradictions, incertitudes, and dead ends—and that understanding can direct scientists toward sounder and more productive studies [30].

As stated earlier, science builds on the works of others. Librarians today must keep intact the record of that chain of development, so that future scholars can consult the preserved collection of literature pertaining to their topics with some certainty that they could in fact document how curiosity led to discovery, how errors were inherited and passed to succeeding generations. They should be able to identify the great individuals as well as the charlatans, read fine writing as well as poor, and know the climate and tenor of the times.

The representative collection must include the full range of materials, both print and nonprint formats. Each format contributes and is necessary to the understanding of the whole. It is not necessary to retain the works of ten authors writing the introduction to genetics or the basic principles of nursing, but it is essential that all points of view be preserved, especially when those points of view are controversial. These factors are basic to decision making in preservation, and they illustrate the complexity of that process.

The criteria governing selection for preservation should be codified in a written policy manual and should be directly related to collecting levels and the interests of the library in the subject. It is also important to determine the role of the library vis-à-vis its collection, that is, where on the spectrum between the preservation of the historical record for future research and to meet current needs does the library fall?

In addition to their utility in routine preservation activities, these criteria are also useful public relations devices for articulating to the user group the library's preservation policy for appropriate disciplines. The policy may then be refined based on user input.

The general criteria for selection for preservation include the following.

Place of the Item or Group of Items within the Literature of the Discipline

A series of questions may be applied to the item, such as: Is the item a first edition? Does it include the initial demonstration of a technique? Is it of historical importance in some other way? Is there a small number of similar publications of this format, subject, period? Is it a "standard" work according to some authority in the discipline? The economic and artifactual value of an item are additional considerations in determining the place of an item within the literature of the discipline. For periodicals, one should consider the current and past "impact" factor of the overall title, as measured, for example, in the numerous publications of the Institute for Scientific Information (ISI).

Content and Type of Publication

The content of an item is typically comprised of primary material, synthesized material, or a combination of the two. Priority for preservation should be given to items that contain primary material.

The type of publication will have a direct bearing on the preservation decision, as described previously. Research journals that report scholarly results based on extensive scientific investigation would likely receive higher priority for preservation over clinical titles that report clinical information in case study format, though the latter may assume a higher priority in some health care disciplines.

Bibliographic Accessibility of the Title through Major Abstracting and Indexing Services

The decision to include a journal in an indexing source increases access to its contents and also its level of use within a library. Relying on predictable use, these titles might assume a higher priority than titles not included in indexing and abstracting services.

Availability and Regional Commitments

The availability of an individual item through consortial agreements may obviate a local preservation measure, but a library should make certain that the copy available through these agreements has in fact been preserved. By the same token, an item that is uniquely or rarely held may be a primary candidate for preservation treatment to insure its continued availability to other institutions.

Cooperative resource-sharing arrangements may have indicators in local serial control records that commit the local institution to maintain a particular title for the consortium. In a similar way, the Research Libraries Group has assigned Primary Collecting Responsibility (PCR) designations to institutions within the consortium. These assignments should be reflected in preservation priority statements and in decision making. NLM has assumed PCR for all RLG Medical and Health Sciences Conspectus areas for which the NLM collection is the only collection at level 5.

Continued Relevance of the Title to the Actual or Potential Needs of Research, Clinical, or Educational Programs of the User Group

Did the item in hand enter the collection for a specific purpose or group, such as a research center, an academic program, a training grant, which no longer exists? If an item is now of purely historical interest, it will assume a different priority in the preservation queue.

A heavy indicator of potential future use and thus the worthiness of a preservation investment is the degree to which an item or a group of items is used in a local situation. That something was used heavily in the past, however, should be interpreted only as a guide for the future.

Quality

The quality of an item can best be determined by weighing several subjective factors collectively, such as its sponsorship; degree of scholarship; its reviewing or refereeing policy; the reputations of the publisher, the editorial board, the authors; the quality of article bibliographies. None of these should be the deciding factor alone, but each should be considered as it contributes to or detracts from the overall quality of the item.

Language and Country of Origin

The criteria of language and country of origin are rarely used as sole determinants for preservation in general health sciences library collections, but may have relevance in special collections.

Intellectual satisfaction would dictate that the full range of criteria be considered for each title; practical considerations, however, preclude that level of activity. A library might instead undertake a review of the criteria against the entire collection or segments of it. For such mass efforts, a priority statement should be developed to serve as a guide for deciding upon preservation treatments for large and small collections.

Preservation Priorities Statement

A preservation priorities statement may be incorporated into a broader policies and procedures statement or may be considered separately. Paulson discusses local policy and procedure statements and includes an example of such a statement [31]. In general, these documents should include three elements: introduction, methodology, and priorities and rationale.

Introduction

The introduction is a general description of the library and its user group, special collections, etc. It includes a statement of the preservation status of the collection, especially including information derived from a condition survey; a description of cooperative agreements and an awareness of what other institutions, including NLM, are doing; a definition of the scope of the preservation effort, and any limitations; the governing principles of selection for preservation, including criteria for selection and methods of selection; a description of the budget and funding support for preservation, including grants.

Methodology

This section contains a detailed procedure statement reflecting personnel involved with assignment of authority and responsibility clearly defined.

Priorities and Rationale

A preservation priorities statement should conclude with a detailed statement of priorities, arranged by number with any qualifications by category. In the *National Preservation Plan for the Biomedical Literature* [32], NLM articulated its priorities for microfilming brittle materials in its collection. These priorities are included in Table 11-1.

In lieu of developing a priorities statement at the level of detail reflected in the NLM document, libraries can identify the most pressing preservation needs for materials of long-term value in their institution. These will likely be unique local publications or those which have a very long useful life span. Once the identification task is completed, a short work plan can be drafted and preservation work completed as time and other resources permit.

Underlying the collection development and preservation efforts of libraries and librarians is the concept of use, potential and actual, by the physician, the scholar, the historian, the nurse, the student, the bench scientist. Perhaps not this year, or even this decade, but it is ultimately for their use that collections are built and resources are preserved.

220 *Collection Development and Assessment*

Table 11-1: National Library of Medicine, Priorities for Preservation Microfilming

In 1987, the National library of Medicine (NLM) issued the National Preservation Plan for the Biomedical Literature. That document set forth the priorities for preservation microfilming of brittle serial volumes in the collection. To minimize redundant microfilming, these priorities took into account past and current filming projects by other libraries and the commercial sector. In 1988, additional priorities were developed for microfilming of the brittle monographs in the NLM collection.

Priorities for Preservation Microfilming of Serials:

- Brittle serials indexed in *Index Medicus*.

- Brittle serials in NLM core subjects currently indexed in NLM databases.

- Brittle serials in NLM core subjects currently indexed in other major abstracting and indexing services (e.g., Excerpta Medica, BIOSIS, Chemical Abstracts, Psychological Abstracts).

- Brittle serials which, according to SERHOLD, are unique to NLM.

- Remaining NLM brittle serials in core subjects.

Priorities for Preservation Microfilming of Monographs

The National Library of Medicine monograph collection numbers in excess of 575,000. Of that number, preservation surveys indicate that some 12.8%, representing about 73,000 volumes or 22,080,000 pages, is embrittled and in need of preservation microfilming. The current preservation microfilming contract provides for the microfilming of 35,000,000 pages over a four- year period. The majority of those pages will be devoted to serials. Consequently, a more detailed priority schedule has been developed to provide a structure within which to queue embrittled monographs in the NLM collection for preservation microfilming. As part of NLM's regular preservation program, approximately 4,000 brittle monographs have already been filmed.

Underlying the priority scheme are the following assumptions:

- All embrittled monographs published between 1800 and 1950 in all core collecting areas, as defined in the Collection Development Manual, will be filmed; in addition, embrittled monographs which are historically important but in disciplines which, under modern definitions, may no longer be considered "core" biomedicine, will be filmed.

- The age and condition of the item govern its priority in the microfilming queue.

- Item-by-item preservation microfilming decisions will not be made for monographs, except as noted in 2c below.

- Monographs in the following categories will not be filmed.

    1. Materials which are heavily illustrated in color, pending development of more effective color microfilming or other preservation technology; these titles will, however, be identified and bibliographic records annotated.
    2. Theses and pamphlets, which together include approximately 450,000 items, will not be queued for microfilming until item-level bibliographic control is available.

3. Multiple copies of the same item; only the "best" copy available in the collection will be filmed.
4. Titles for which preservation quality microfilm is already available, either commercially or from another institution.
   N.B. Items in categories 1. and 2. which are in such poor condition that immediate attention is warranted may be queued for preservation microfilming.
- Funding to continue the preservation microfilming program at NLM will be included in future budget requests.

Given the above assumptions, monographs will be filmed in the following order:

Priority 1: Embrittled Monographs Published Between 1801 and 1914.

1a. Monographs published in the United States between 1801 and 1900 in WZ 270 of the National Library of Medicine classification schedule.
1b. All other monographs published between 1801 and 1914.

Materials in this category have been selected for initial microfilm queuing for the following reasons:

- This category contains the highest percentage (48.5%) of brittle monographs within a readily identifiable collection category.
- This category contains the oldest brittle items in the collection.
- These monographs are physically together, allowing for the most efficient personnel and work flow.

Priority 2: Embrittled Monographs Published Between 1914 and 1950.

Modern monographs will be filmed in the following order:

2a. Monographs in Medicine and Related Subjects in classification numbers W through WZ.
2b. Monographs in Preclinical Sciences in classification number QS through QZ.
2c. Monographs in Library of Congress classification numbers which are regarded, currently or historically, as important to core biomedicine. Within category 2c, the initial filming effort will focus on those aspects of these subjects which are collected comprehensively.

Queuing for preservation microfilming using a priority scheme based on the NLM and LC classification schedules is proposed for the following reasons:

- embrittled modern monographs in core biomedicine will be filmed first;
- the number of core biomedical titles diminishes with each category, maximizing the number of large segments of the collection which can be identified for preservation microfilming, and minimizing the number of items for which item-by-item decisions must be made;
- filmed titles will be grouped by subject, facilitating subject access by users.

Whether a library begins a preservation effort by restoring some broken spines, or filming a few major journals, or mounting a full-blown preservation program, the principles are the same. The policies developed for building the library's collection must form the basis for the decisions to select the materials to be preserved. Since all materials cannot, and, indeed, should not be retained, a balance must be maintained between the needs of current users and the preservation of materials that will be useful and needed over time.

The criteria outlined previously illustrate the principles on which selection for preservation in the health sciences should be based. They should be used in conjunction with the library's individual programs and disciplines. All processes, from basic weeding of the collection through building and preserving its components, must reflect some consideration beyond local demands by including regional and national preservation efforts. Policies and procedures should not be promulgated in a vacuum, but rather in consultation with NLM and other institutions, and with an awareness of the activities of others in this vital area.

The *National Preservation Plan for the Biomedical Literature* is based on the recognized need to preserve all of the important biomedical literature held by health sciences libraries in this country. Local decisions can, therefore, have a significant impact on the national effort. The scholarly record for biomedicine includes substantial resources held in institutions outside of NLM, and these resources constitute a portion of the nation's heritage in health care. A coordinated and cooperative effort will be needed if today's medical libraries, as a group, are to meet the demands of the future.

References

1. Holmes OW. Medical essays, 1842-1882. Boston: Houghton Mifflin, 1891:400.
2. Abelson PH. Brittle books and journals. Science 1987 Oct 30;238(4827):595.
3. Clark L, ed. Guide to review of library collections: preservation, storage, and withdrawal. Chicago: American Library Association, 1991. (Collection management and development guides, no. 5.)
4. Slote S. Weeding library collections. 3rd ed. Littleton, CO: Libraries Unlimited, 1989.
5. Hazen DC. Collection development, collection management, and preservation. Libr Res Tech Serv 1982 Jan/Mar;26(1):6-10.
6. Walker G. Preserving the intellectual content of deteriorated library materials. In: Morrow CC. The preservation challenge: a guide to conserving library materials. White Plains, NY: Knowledge Industry, 1983:95-101.
7. Kirkpatrick BA. Preservation activities and needs in U.S. biomedical libraries: a status report. Bull Med Libr Assoc 1989 Jul;77(3)276-83.
8. Atkinson RW. Selection for preservation: a materialistic approach. Libr Res Tech Serv 1986 Oct/Dec;30(4):341-53.

9. The RLG Conspectus on-line user's manual. Stanford, CA: Research Libraries Group, 1987.

10. Child MS. Further thoughts on "Selection for preservation: a materialistic approach." Libr Res Tech Serv 1986 Oct/Dec;30(4):354-62.

11. Bagnall RS, Harris CL. Involving scholars in preservation decisions: the case of the classicists. J Acad Libr 1987 Jul;13(3):140-6.

12. Byrnes MM, ed. Symposium: Preservation of the biomedical literature. Bull Med Libr Assoc 1989 Jul;77(3):256-98.

13. DeBakey L, DeBakey S. Our silent enemy: ashes in our libraries. Bull Med Libr Assoc 1989 Jul;77(3):258-68.

14. Ibid., 259.

15. Byrnes MM. Preservation of the biomedical literature: an overview. Bull Med Libr Assoc 1989 Jul;77(3):269-75.

16. Ibid., 274.

17. Kirkpatrick, op. cit., 283.

18. Richards DT, McClure LW. Selection for preservation: considerations for the health sciences. Bull Med Libr Assoc 1989 Jul;77(3):284-92.

19. Paulson BA. Developing a preservation policy and procedure statement for a health sciences library. Bull Med Libr Assoc 1989 Jul;77(3):293-8.

20. Carr E. Symposium: weeding the medical library: medical school libraries. Bull Med Libr Assoc 1952 Apr;40(2):162-3.

21. Murphy MA. Medical school libraries. Bull Med Libr Assoc 1952 Apr;40(2):164-5.

22. Felter JW. Weeding the special hospital library. Bull Med Libr Assoc 1952 Apr;40(2):165-6.

23. Reilley JM. On weeding an association library. Bull Med Libr Assoc 1952 Apr;40(2):166-8.

24. Marshall ML. Pamphlet weeding. Bull Med Libr Assoc 1952 Apr;40(2):168-9.

25. Duffield P. Discarding sets of medical books. Bull Med Libr Assoc 1953 Oct;41(4):361-4.

26. Ibid., 362-3.

27. Meckel CL. Bigger or better collections? Bull Med Libr Assoc 1953 Oct;41(4):365-8.

28. Patterson MA. Some practical aspects of medical society library operation: a symposium. Preserve or discard? A problem in librarianship. Bull Med Libr Assoc 1958 Jan;46(1):45-9.

29. Doe J. Best books in medicine. Bull Med Libr Assoc 1953 Jan;41(1):78-9.

30. DeBakey L. Book-burning in our medical libraries: prevention or palliation? Am J Cardiol 1988 Sept 1;62(7):459.

31. Paulson, op. cit.

32. National Library of Medicine. National preservation plan for the biomedical literature. Bethesda, MD: National Library of Medicine, Jan 1988.

12

Research Questions and Future Issues in Collection Development

"Everyone knows that in research there are no final answers, only insights that allow one to formulate new questions."

S. E. Luria

The Medical Library Association promotes and supports research activities by health sciences librarians. Two goals within the association's research policy statement are particularly relevant.

- Use the health information science knowledge base to design, develop, and market new health information systems and services, including those that integrate scientific literature with other types of health-related information.

- Add to the health information science knowledge base by carrying out research that is broadly relevant to the organization, delivery, use, and impact of information on health care, biomedical research, and health professionals' education [1].

The field of collection development and management offers fertile ground for research, as there are many gaps in knowledge about the literature of medicine and its use. Furthermore, the concept of nonprint "literature" has expanded to encompass the broader context of information resources and knowledge bases. Collection management is evolving into knowledge management [2].

Librarians make decisions about collections—what to purchase and what not to purchase, when to acquire materials locally and when to use electronic access, how to allocate funds, what to keep and what to discard, which resources to point users to through networks and which to ignore. Some claim these decisions are primarily an art; others argue that they are, or should be, grounded in scientific methods. All would agree, however, that good decisions are based on a broad knowledge of the health sciences literature and of user needs. The depth and extent of their knowledge will influence how effectively librarians make decisions about health sciences collections. Outlined in this chapter are some of the areas in which further research is needed to expand the base of knowledge and some of the issues libraries will be facing.

Research Questions

Literature Analysis

Published literature can be analyzed in many ways. Bibliometric studies examine the relationships among publications. They look at how the literature of a given discipline or subspecialty is distributed in the journal literature. It may be scattered throughout a broad array of journals or concentrated in a few highly specialized publications. Such analysis can demonstrate the interdependence of disciplines. When the literature of one field is isolated from that of another, seemingly unrelated field, scientists may fail to recognize important relationships or the applicability of knowledge in another field to a set of problems in their own specialty [3]. The challenge is how to structure the literature so that such potential relationships can be discerned. Bradford long ago introduced the concept of scattering, demonstrating that a predictable proportion of the relevant literature in any given field would be concentrated in a small number of journals [4]. While many studies based on these laws of scattering have followed, biomedical disciplines as well as their literature are constantly changing and further research could reach new conclusions. The growth of widespread electronic communication, personal publishing, and electronic journals introduced new complexities in disseminating biomedical knowledge and practice.

Citation analysis is another form of bibliometric research. Since the inception of citation indexing, which traces the path of references authors make to each other's (or their own) published work, studies recording and analyzing the patterns of citation have abounded [5-6]. *Current Contents* frequently publishes articles tracing the citation history of seminal articles and scientific advances. The weekly essays are collected and published separately [7]. Such studies may be used to distill the literature and identify key papers in a specialized field. They may also be used to support claims that an individual investigator has contributed substantially to the growth of knowledge. Those who use citation data in making decisions for hiring or promoting faculty argue that if the individual's work is cited, it must be useful or important. Opinions about the validity of citation analysis differ [8-11]. While controversy will continue over how valid particular applications may be, citation research nevertheless remains a useful tool for analyzing the scientific literature if the limitations are understood and care is taken in research design [12].

Publishing Trends

Akin to literature analysis, but broader in focus, the study of biomedical publishing can contribute to a better understanding of how information is disseminated and the factors that make dissemination effective. The early growth of biomedical literature has received considerable study [13-14]. A clear understanding of the past provides insights into the practices of the present. Much is left to be learned regarding the relationship of specific publications to the evolution of biomedicine and related health fields. What is the relationship between the rise and fall of journals and how biomedical research is conducted and supported? What are the causes and results of specialization and subspecialization in journals—the phenomena of branching and twigging? What is the impact of the opposite but parallel trend toward more interdisciplinary research? How has responsibility for publishing changed and what effect have those changes had on the dissemination of information? What roles are played by commercial publishers, scholarly organizations, academic institutions, and private industry in making available the results of research and information related to clinical practice?

The emergence of electronic publishing raises a host of new questions. How will traditional publications be affected by new modes of communication? There is no question that the nature of the relationships between publishers, vendors, libraries, and researchers or clinicians are changing and will continue to change; but in what ways? Collaborative ventures, such as Red Sage and TULIP, between libraries, communication specialists, and publishers promise quicker, easier access to full-text journal content [15-17].

Use of Information

How information is sought and used, and how well it meets the needs of those who use or don't use it, are questions that lie at the heart of health sciences librarianship. To the extent that the published literature remains a primary source for established medical knowledge, such questions will also be central to collection development. At least one study has suggested that health sciences libraries do not succeed very well in selecting books that will be used [18]. In addition to describing the structure of the literature, citation analysis can also be used to study how the literature is used. The various health professions—physicians, dentists, nurses, pharmacists, veterinarians, and others—differ in the extent to which they rely on published information. They also differ in the importance they attribute to various types of literature, such as books, reviews, research journals, practical articles, reports of meetings, or even dissertations. The needs of physicians in training are not the same as those of experienced clinicians. Even first year medical students have different needs than fourth year students. Practitioners require different types of information than researchers. How do health professionals keep current in their fields; does the literature serve their needs well? Some have argued that medical journals in their present form do not present the kind of information needed by clinicians [19].

The trend in biomedical journals toward requiring structured abstracts is intended to guarantee the reader a certain amount and type of information condensed from the article. For users of electronic retrieval systems who judge the usefulness of articles by reading the abstract, structured summaries should be especially valuable. But do they serve their purpose? To what extent do readers rely solely on information in the abstract, never consulting the full articles? Do they make clinical decisions from this data? What are the consequences?

The role of published literature in the dissemination and acceptance of new knowledge and practice must be investigated. How do clinicians learn about new diagnostic methods, new therapies, new drugs, new instrumentation, or even new management techniques? What convinces them to incorporate such information into their own practice? How is the health practitioner or biomedical researcher affected by the ways they are able to access published information; how important is the convenience factor in selecting what publications they read or consult? To what extent has language been a barrier to the dissemination of information from one country to another? These questions are of more than academic interest. Information may have financial impact: the cost of diagnostic or therapeutic procedures, or time spent in the hospital; patient care impact: effectiveness of clinical decisions; legal impact: whether the physician is following currently accepted practice standards. Some work has been done in these areas, but much more needs to be known [20-24].

With encouragement from the National Library of Medicine and the health sciences library community in general, health professionals are increasingly using a variety of electronic sources to search the literature themselves. Has this changed the extent to which they turn to the literature to solve clinical problems? Have concerns about litigation affected the patterns of literature use?

Another direction for research is determining which literature actually gets used and why. Studies of interlibrary loan handled through the National Library of Medicine's DOCLINE system indicate that only a small proportion of the published articles ever get requested through interlibrary loan [25]. Is this also true of the use of individual library collections? Do collections in health sciences libraries with a primary purpose of providing a working collection show a higher proportion of articles used than collections in research libraries? Many libraries look at the extent to which specific journal titles in their collections are used, but very little is known about the fate of individual articles. Electronic full-text databases and electronic journals will begin to provide some data for study. Such information may be useful in making future decisions about the structure of information delivery systems and new publication formats.

Quality

Much remains to be studied regarding the quality of published literature. How accurate is the information published in books and journals; to what degree has scientific inaccuracy, whether it is the result of fraud or merely sloppiness in research, crept into the literature? What is the role of peer review and how effective is it in judging quality and eliminating chaff? How will peer review change in an environment of universal electronic communication, where comments and critiques are interactive and immediate, and reviewers may be self-selected? What will be the barriers to publishing unpopular theories or unorthodox therapies? How do the decisions of the local library about what journals and books to acquire, or the decisions of the National Library of Medicine or other publishers about what to include in indexes such as MEDLINE, serve as quality filters? Is such filtering effective in pointing the user to the best information or do they only succeed in reducing the quantity to a more manageable size?

Economics

The economics of biomedical publishing arouses strong sentiments among librarians and publishers alike. Beyond the rhetoric and blame-pointing regarding rising journal prices, differential charges, and copyright restrictions lie serious questions deserving thorough study. Costs associated with information dissemination, whether by commercial publisher, professional society, or academic institution, need to be more carefully analyzed. Electronic alternatives to paper publications pose many additional questions, not only about how the information will be disseminated and in what form, but how it will be paid for, and by whom. These are issues that require practical economic as well as policy decisions. To aid in decision making and to evaluate the effect of new technology on the price of information will require rigorous data gathering and research.

Changes in the cost of published materials and changes in the mode of access to information have profound effects on budgeting in libraries. These changes affect how costs are allocated for materials and access. An understanding of how library budgets for collections and access have evolved over time would provide those struggling with current problems a historical perspective that could be useful, or at least comforting.

The opportunities for investigation are endless. Whether topics for doctoral dissertations, research grants, or more limited individual projects, better information should lead to greater understanding and a more rational approach to collection development—a balance between serendipity and science.

Future Issues in Collection Development

The nature of libraries is changing rapidly, driven or enabled by technology, depending on one's point of view. Many of the issues mentioned here affect libraries of all types and will not be dealt with in detail. However, because the biomedical sciences are intensely dependent on information and are often in the forefront of technological innovation, the impact may be felt sooner in health sciences libraries.

Library as Information Center

Much talk and writing has occurred over the past decade and more, predicting the paperless society, the library without walls, and the electronic library. The term virtual library, now in vogue, denotes the invisibility of physical perimeters between libraries and information sources worldwide; it also implies an infinite capacity for expanded resources.

Rapid national and international network communication and the ability to transmit high-quality images, as well as text, will remove the physical barriers to instantaneous transmission of documents. Journals, as static compilations of individual articles, may begin to fade, while the least publishable unit—perhaps the article, perhaps an abstract, or perhaps some as yet undefined form—may exist independently in a database for individualized retrieval. What will be role of individual library collections in this environment? Increasingly, libraries will need to determine not only what information to make available, but in what format and how it will be distributed to those who need it. Local collections are likely to shrink and users will rely on other means of distribution—collections in other libraries, central clearinghouses or data banks, direct from publisher, and even direct from author.

As the means of publication and distribution change, libraries will emphasize the role of aiding the user in finding the needed information through an increasingly complex universe of sources. In an environment of constant, rapid, and sometimes dramatic technological advances, the possible will remain beyond the reach of most users' equipment, knowledge, and patience. In addition to their roles as navigators, advisors, and teachers, librarians must take responsibility for seeing that the structure of information in electronic formats and the design of systems by which that knowledge is disseminated are truly responsive to the users' needs. This is a role librarians have played somewhat weakly in the past. The focus of the future will be less on developing collections and more on delivering the information effectively.

New Technology

Graphical interfaces between user and text or data should continue to improve. Librarians must take an active role in developing the methods by which full text can be most effectively searched to meet a variety of user needs. The methods used for retrieval at the level of a book, article, or even abstract, are not necessarily optimal for searching large volumes of text or graphical material.

In addition to the growth of electronic publishing, advances in optical storage technology will have an impact on library collections. Conversion of print collections to optical storage media may offer alternatives to expanded buildings or storage facilities, while preserving the economies of local access. Costs and feasibility will have to be weighed against costs of access to the same sources through a vendor or centralized service. The costs of conversion and availability of satisfactory and affordable retrieval software will be major factors. Digital imaging techniques permitting electronic delivery and high quality display of page images will remove barriers to effective network transmission of full text.

Publishing

The number of electronic journals is growing rapidly. The American Chemical Society (ACS), through its Chemical Journals Online, has made full text of the last ten years of twenty ACS journals, as well as those of a number of commercial publishers accessible. While these and most journals currently available in electronic form also have a print counterpart, journals that are totally electronic are entering the market. The collaborative project of the American Association for the Advancement of Science (AAAS) and OCLC resulted in the first fully electronic medical journal, the *Online Journal of Current Clinical Trials*. This pioneer effort, initiated in 1992, contained peer reviewed content and offered a graphical interface and use of hypertext to access figures, tables, and references. In addition, it could provide for online alerts to letters, rebuttals, and retractions. The software permitted multiple modes of access. While this publication had a rocky start and a commercial publisher eventually replaced AAAS as a collaborator with OCLC, it demonstrated some of the capabilities that electronic publications can offer over print. The Association of Computing Machinery plans to convert its journals to an entirely electronic form of communication. As electronic journals become more prevalent, libraries will be challenged to define their role with respect to acquiring, making accessible to users, maintaining, and preserving.

If institutions, especially universities, move toward taking more control over the publishing output of their own faculty, libraries may find new roles as publishers or as participants in the publishing process. On-demand publishing and self-publishing may change the way knowledge is packaged, raising questions about what constitutes a publication, how the peer review process is handled, and the impact on quality control.

The key functions of the scientific journal, in order of importance as proposed by Schaffner, are building a collective knowledge base, communicating information, validating the quality of research, distributing rewards, and building scientific communities [26]. Some functions, such as creating a collective knowledge base for the public record, and the peer review process that maintains standards and serves as a quality filter, may not adapt readily into the electronic environment, while other functions, such as information sharing through informal communication, have already been transformed by new technology. Schaffner argues that authors must be confident that electronic journals serve as a reliable source of knowledge and that the information content conveyed by the current formal structure of journal articles must not be lost in the new age of electronic publication.

Electronic publishing may not only speed the process of publication but will allow authors to include more data and information not now available to reviewers or readers because of space restrictions in journals. This process may lead to greater interaction between authors and readers: the electronically published report is only the first step, followed by criticism, revisions, comments, and abstracts of related articles [27].

Numerous issues have been raised by those who are facing both the potential and the challenge of electronic publishing in the sciences [28-30]:

- How will control over quality be maintained?
- Will peer review still take place, and if so, how?
- How will public access be assured?
- How will authorship be attributed and credit assigned in an interactive environment?
- How will intellectual property rights be defined and maintained?
- How will distribution be controlled?
- Who will be responsible for maintaining the authenticity of content?
- How will continued retrievability be assured?
- How will the development of knowledge be archived and preserved for future scientific work?

LaPorte et al. speak optimistically of a "Global Health Information Server" which will permit the scientific community ". . . to redesign the mode of information transfer—the journal article itself." They argue that the concepts of "article," "paper," and "publication" should die and be replaced by new forms of research communications[31].

Copyright

Issues related to ownership of intellectual property and the legitimate but sometimes conflicting rights of publishers, authors, libraries, and users of information will continue to plague those who create the laws and those who interpret them. Solutions will not come easily or soon. As Bennett has pointed out, users will have many choices for acquiring information in the future, and the library will be only one of them. "What will distinguish the digital library from all other providers of digital information...will be the way in which it assists readers in exercising their fair use rights—and in advancing the Constitutional purpose of the copyright law" [32].

Preservation

Atkinson speaks eloquently of the dangers of what he terms "text mutability":

> It is becoming clear...that it is not only the quantity and flow of information, but also its fragility, its perishability, which will characterize the online era. It is becoming clear that we can purchase the ability to manipulate information only at the expense of its stability— at the expense...of the information's own history [33].

He argues for the unique role of libraries "to select, stabilize, protect and provide access to significant or representative graphic texts," regardless of format [34]. This mission will constitute an enormous challenge to libraries in the coming years.

Economics of Information

Who would dare to say what scientific publishing will look like in even as short a time as ten years? The journal has not vanished as predicted in the past. Every month publishers announce new journals; every year *Index Medicus* grows bigger. Yet the struggle over ever-increasing prices intensifies and health science libraries are paring their collections further, year after year. This paring is not necessarily a bad thing. No one has yet demonstrated that smaller collections have adversely affected medical education, patient care, or biomedical research. If the trend continues, however, will collections across the country look more uniform and will access to very specialized or esoteric literature be lost?

Budget restrictions will drive most libraries to emphasize acquiring materials at the time of need, replacing the historical practice of purchasing in anticipation of need. Retrospective collections will be fewer, increasing the burden on large research libraries to share their resources.

Electronic publication is beginning to take a greater hold—whether for local access on CD-ROMs and floppy disks or through network access to remote vendors or publishers. Electronic publishing produces a tangle of economic issues related to copyright ownership, intellectual property rights, cost of production, control and pricing of telecommunications, use charges, and expense of equipment to access, retrieve, and manipulate electronic information. As the technology advances, hardware and software requirements change. Upgrades necessary to take advantage of new forms of distribution and display add to the cost of access. Library budgets will need to reflect the changed information environment, taking account of the greater reliance on access to external resources. "Collection" funds will be directed to the best source of information, which may not be the local print collection. These issues sharpen the need for an institutional information policy that will help guide decisions. Decisions will be made in a broader context, involving players other than the library. Computer and information technology specialists, network managers, and the library's constituent groups will be partners in determining how scarce resources will be allocated to making information of many kinds available in the institution.

And Beyond

The environment for libraries in general and collections in particular is changing rapidly. This final chapter has touched upon some of the trends and issues that are affecting the library's role in managing health sciences information. While the future of collection development is far from clear, any update of this work is likely to take a radically different form.

References

1. Using scientific evidence to improve information practice: the research policy statement of the Medical Library Association. Chicago: Medical Library Association, [1995]: 6-7.

2. Lucier RE. Towards a knowledge management environment: a strategic framework. EDUCOM Rev 1992 Nov/Dec; 27(6): 24-31.

3. Swanson DR. Two medical literatures that are logically but not bibliographically connected. JASIS Jul 1987: 38(4):228-233.

4. Bradford SC. Documentation. Washington, DC: Public Affairs Press, 1950: 110-20.

5. Garfield E. Citation indexing—its theory and application in science, technology, and humanities. New York: John Wiley, 1979.

6. Garfield E. Citation analysis as a tool in journal evaluation. Science 1972 Nov 3; 178(60): 471-9.

7. Garfield E. Essays of an information scientist. Philadelphia: ISI Press, v.1-15, 1962-93.

8. Barlup J. Mechanization of library procedures in the medium-sized medical library. VII. Relevancy of cited articles in citation indexing. Bull Med Libr Assoc 1969 Jul; 57(3):260-3.

9. Brodman E. Choosing physiology journals. Bull Med Libr Assoc 1944 Oct; 32(4): 479-83.

10. Margolis J. Citation indexing and evaluation of scientific papers. Science 1967 Mar 10; 155(767):1213-9.

11. Smith LC. Citation analysis. Libr Trends 1981 Summer; 30(1): 83-106.

12. Peritz BC. On the objectives of the citation analysis: problems of theory and method. J Amer Soc Inf Sci 1992 Jul; 43(6):448-51.

13. Brodman E. The development of medical bibliography. Baltimore: Medical Library Association, 1954.

14. Kronick DA. A history of scientific and technical periodicals: the origins and development of the scientific and technical press, 1665-1790. 2nd ed. Metuchen, NJ: Scarecrow Press, 1976.

15. DeLoughry TJ. University of California's Red Sage project electronic document delivery. Chron Higher Educ 1993 Apr 7;39(31):A19.

16. Lucier RE, Badger RC. Red Sage project. Ser Libr 1994; 24(3/4):129-34.

17. Willis K, Alexander K, Gosling WA, Peters GR Jr, et al. TULIP—the university licensing program: experiences at the University of Michigan. Ser Rev 1994 Fall;20(3):39-47.

18. Fenske RE. Evaluation of monograph selection in a health sciences library. Bull Med Libr Assoc 1994 Jul;82(3):265-70.

19. Haynes BR. Loose connections between peer-reviewed clinical journals and clinical practices. Ann Intern Med 1990 Nov 1; 113(9):724-8.

20. Gorman PN, Ash J, Wykoff L. Can primary care physicians' questions be answered using the medical literature? Bull Med Libr Assoc 1994 Apr; 82(2):140-6.

21. Klein MS, Ross FV, Adams DL, Gilbert CM. Effect of online literature searching on length of stay and patient care costs. Acad Med 1994 Jun;69(6):489-95.

22. Marshall JG. The impact of the hospital library on clinical decision making: the Rochester study. Bull Med Libr Assoc 1992 Apr;80(2):169-78.

23. Manning PR, Lee PV, Clintworth WA, Denson TA, et al. Changing prescribing practices through individual continuing education. JAMA 1986 Jul 11;256(2):230-2.

24. Manning PR, Lee PV, Denson TA, Gilman NJ. Determining educational needs in the physician's office. JAMA 1980 Sep 5;244(10):1112-5.

25. Lacroix EM. Interlibrary loan in U.S. health sciences libraries: journal article use. Bull Med Libr Assoc 1994 Oct;82(4):363-8.

26. Schaffner AC. The future of scientific journals: lessons from the past. Info Tech Libr 1994 Dec; 13(4): 239-47.

27. Judson HF. Structural transformations of the sciences and the end of peer review. JAMA 1994 Jul 13; 272(2):92-4.

28. Kassirer JP, Angell M. The Internet and the *Journal*. New Engl J Med 1995 Jun 22;332(25):1709-10.

29. Winograd S, Zare RN. "Wired" science or whither the printed page? Science 1995 Aug 4;269(5224):615.

30. Cochenour D, Moothart T. Relying on the kindness of strangers: archiving electronic journals on Gopher. Ser Rev 1995 Spring;21(1):67-76.

31. LaPorte RE, Marler E, Akazawa S, Sauer F, et al. The death of biomedical journals. Brit Med J 1995 May 27;310(6991):1387-90.

32. Bennett S. The copyright challenge: strengthening the public interest in the digital age. Libr J 1994 Nov 15;119(19):34-7.

33. Atkinson R. Text mutability and collection administration. Libr Acq Pract Theory 1990; 14(4):355-8.

34. Ibid., 356.

Appendix A

Examples from Collection Development Policies

The examples which follow are taken from Collection Development Policies for Health Sciences Libraries, compiled by David H. Morse and Daniel T. Richards (Chicago: Medical Library Association, 1992). The arrangement of the examples follows the outline for a collection development policy suggested in Chapter 4: Policies and Criteria.

EXAMPLE OF AN INSTITUTIONAL MISSION STATEMENT:

SOUTHERN ILLINOIS UNIVERSITY (SPRINGFIELD, IL)
MEDICAL LIBRARY

2. Institutional Mission, Goals, and Relationships
   2.1 School of Medicine
      The mission of the Southern Illinois University School of Medicine is to assist the people of central and southern Illinois in meeting their present and future health care needs through education and research. The goals of the School are:

    * to offer programs in undergraduate, graduate, and continuing medical education responsive to advances in medical knowledge, skills, and technology and to the health care needs of this region;
    * to provide service to the region through tertiary patient care facilities and specialists, by support of health care delivery systems, and by contributions to programs in public education and allied health education;
    * to develop and maintain research into the sciences basic to medicine and the clinical sciences which include studies related to the cultural and behavioral aspects of medicine and the medical education process as well as methods of health care delivery.

   2.2 Department of Information and Communication Science and the Medical Library
      The Department of Information and Communication Sciences in the academic unit with the mission to identify and meet the information needs of School of Medicine students, faculty, and staff through education and research activities relating to the acquisition, organization, storage, dissemination, and evaluation of information resources. The Medical Library is the administrative unit with the mission to select, acquire, organize, store, provide, and utilize information resources, regardless of format, to meet the information needs of School of Medicine personnel for purposes of education, research, administration, and patient care. The Medical Library serves an extended audience through networking arrangements described below.

EXAMPLE OF A COOPERATIVE PROGRAMS STATEMENT:

UNIVERSITY OF MICHIGAN (ANN ARBOR, MI)
ALFRED TAUBMAN MEDICAL LIBRARY

IX. COOPERATION AND RESOURCE SHARING

The University Library System

The Alfred Taubman Medical Library is a divisional library within the University Library system. It is the major library in a cluster of health science libraries, which also includes the Dentistry and Public Health libraries. The health science libraries work closely together, sharing information prior to ordering or canceling journal subscriptions, especially in areas of overlapping interest.

Other units within the University Library system have strongly related collections. Materials in the biological sciences, especially at the cellular and molecular level, and in organic chemistry and medicinal chemistry are found in the Natural Science/Chemistry Libraries. Bioengineering materials are found in the Engineering Library. Many works in the social sciences and publications related to social and community services are in the Social Work Library. Students and faculty of the School of Nursing often use this collection. The Graduate Library has the most comprehensive collection in psychology. Cooperative activities in collection development among these libraries are less formal than among the health sciences libraries, but information is frequently exchanged. Duplication, especially of journal subscriptions, is minimized, but not avoided altogether. Important and heavily used titles may be found in more than one library.

Other campus libraries

Outside the University Library system are other libraries with collections that relate in some way to the medical library. The Law Library acquires very little in medical ethics and forensic medicine but gives considerable attention to psychiatry and the law. The Bentley Historical Library is the official archives for the University and contains many items pertaining to the history of the Medical School and to the development of medicine in Michigan.

Some small libraries are associated with separate institutes on campus. Examples are the Institute of Gerontology, the Burn Center, and the Mental Health Research Institute. The primary purpose of these very specialized collections is to serve the institute staff. While useful for their own clientele and occasionally for referral, these collections rarely affect acquisition decisions for the Taubman Library.

The Regional Medical Library Program

The Regional Medical Library Program is intended to provide health science practitioners, investigators, educators, and administrators in the United States with timely, convenient access to health care and biomedical information resources. The program is coordinated by the National Library of Medicine and is carried out through a nationwide network of more than 3,000 health science libraries and information centers. The network includes seven Regional Medical Libraries. The Taubman Medical Library is a resource library in the Greater Midwest Regional Medical Library Network (Region 3). Through this network the library has access to the holdings of medical libraries throughout the country. A union list of monographs and audiovisuals for Region 3 provides information for borrowing books not available at Taubman. Both regional and national union lists of serials give locations for periodicals in the health sciences. A newly established communications network, DOCLINE, will make borrowing among health science libraries more efficient in the future.

Research Libraries Group

The Research Libraries Group (RLG) is a corporation owned by major research institutions in the United States. RLG is dedicated to improving the management of information resources through a series of cooperative programs:

Research Libraries Information Network (RLIN)
Shared Resources Program
Collection Management and Development Program
Materials Preservation Program.

The intent of RLG programs is to support the transition from locally self-sufficient and independently comprehensive collections to a system of interdependencies that will improve the ability of member libraries to serve the research needs of their constituents.

The Shared Resources Program provides member libraries and their clientele ready access to the holdings of other RLG libraries. It is supported by RLIN, which provides location information and transmits requests electronically to lending institutions.

The purpose of the Collection Management and Development Program is to minimize duplicative purchasing of particular categories of material, while simultaneously ensuring that all materials of research value in designated fields will be acquired by at least one member institution, or, by agreement, by another institution.

The RLG Conspectus is a collection evaluation tool that permits member libraries to survey the existing strengths and current collecting interests of other participating institutions. Available both in paper copy and online, the conspectus is arranged by broad subject divisions, and within each division by more specific subtopics. Libraries undertaking the assessment of their collections use standard codes to describe the relative strengths of their existing collections and the level at which they are currently acquiring material in each area. Language codes indicate language coverage and notes highlight special features.

EXAMPLE OF A GENERAL DESCRIPTION OF THE COLLECTION:

UNIVERSITY OF ARIZONA (TUCSON, AZ)
ARIZONA HEALTH SCIENCES LIBRARY

Overview of the Collection

The AHS Library generally collects at the research and instructional support levels. It provides major source materials adequate for dissertation preparation, and independent research; and it includes a wide selection of scholarly works and specialized monographs, major indexing and abstracting tools, and other reference works.

As the AHS Library is the only medical resource library in the state, it strives to collect materials published by the various health-related agencies in Arizona, and, on a broader level, in the Southwestern region. In view of the recent College of Medicine proposal to establish a program to study the history of medicine focusing on the development and practice of medicine in the Southwest, the AHS Library will play a major role in acquiring and preserving historic and classic works of importance to support this program effectively.

Recent developments also indicate that archival materials and historical documents related to the College of Nursing will be obtained on a continuing basis.

The AHS Library will maintain excellence in its collection in the areas including nursing, psychiatry, pharmacology, neurology, general medicine, orthopedics, pediatrics, cardiology, cancer research, and biochemistry. In support of the anticipated programs outlined in "Vision 2000," College of Medicine's strategic plan for 1991-1996 (rev. draft . Aug. 27, 1991), the Library will strengthen such areas as emergency medicine, epidemiology, rehabilitation, public health, and health services research. Other focus areas that need to be developed include biotechnology, transplantation, patient education, and information technology.

EXAMPLE OF A COLLECTION DESCRIPTION FOR NURSING:

COLUMBIA UNIVERSITY (NEW YORK, NY)
AUGUSTUS C. LONG HEALTH SCIENCES LIBRARY

II. DESCRIPTION OF COLLECTION

The Health Sciences Library has long had a strong commitment to the nursing sciences and its holdings are extensive. The Library collects English language nursing books to the research level including all basic reference works and a wide selection of monographs, textbooks, and periodicals in the major branches of nursing. In addition to these printed sources, the Media Center has a large number of items of interest to the School of Nursing. Especially strong audiovisual collections exist for nursing ethics, nurse midwifery, and nursing in the medical specialties. The Library maintains a standing order to receive all publications of the National League for Nursing.

Nursing is considered one of the Library's core subjects for collecting. Because of the importance of nursing education in the CPMC, the large population of nursing students, and the numerous graduate programs, the intent is to develop a substantial research collection from the nursing literature. The collection includes materials in all areas of nursing science with current collecting activity concentrating on the following:

NURSE CLINICIANS	NURSING ETHICS
NURSE PRACTITIONERS	NURSING JURISPRUDENCE
NURSING AS A PROFESSION	NURSING RESEARCH
NURSING ECONOMICS	NURSING TECHNIQUES
NURSING EDUCATION	PSYCHOLOGICAL ASPECTS
	OF NURSING

as well as the several specialties of nursing both within the field of nursing and as nursing is practiced within the medical specialties, e.g. PSYCHIATRIC NURSING, ONCOLOGY NURSING, COMMUNITY HEALTH NURSING, MATERNAL-CHILD HEALTH NURSING, MEDICAL-SURGICAL NURSING.

Policy governing collecting for the History of Nursing is reflected in the Rare Books and Special Collections policy statement for the Health Sciences Library.

Similarly, policy related to the collection of audiovisual and microcomputer software is included in the policy statement covering those materials.

EXAMPLE OF AN EXCERPT FROM A DEFINITIONS SECTION:

COLUMBIA UNIVERSITY (NEW YORK, NY)
AUGUSTUS C. LONG HEALTH SCIENCES LIBRARY

I. LEVELS OF COVERAGE

The following five levels define the scope and strength of collections in specific subject areas. Each succeeding level of collecting is presumed to be inclusive of those which precede it. The definitions are based upon those developed by the Research Libraries Group for its conspectus program.

> **Minimal level:** A collection in which very few selections are made beyond a representative textbook, a single dictionary, and a single periodical subscription.

> **Basic Information level:** A highly selective collection which serves to introduce and define a subject, and to indicate the varieties of materials available elsewhere. It includes a representative selection of dictionaries, encyclopedias, historical surveys, bibliographies, and handbooks. It contains selected editions of textbooks and monographs and the periodicals cited in the Brandon-Hill list. This collection is not sufficiently intensive to support course work or independent study in the subject.

> **Instructional support level:** A selective collection which is adequate to support undergraduate and most graduate instruction, sustained independent study within a curriculum and health care in a hospital or clinical setting; that is, a collection which is adequate to maintain knowledge of a subject required for limited or generalized purposes, but a collection of less than research intensity. It includes for the subject its major reference tools, the significant indexing and abstracting services, a broad selection of major textbooks, monographs, and government documents, and a wide range of basic periodicals, including at least 25 percent of the English language titles pertinent to the subject which are included in *List of Journals Indexed in Index Medicus*. Materials in languages other than English are seldom included and older or superseded materials are not usually retained for historical research.

> **Research level:** A collection which contains the major published source materials required for dissertations and independent research, including specialized reference tools, conference proceedings, professional society publications, technical reports, government documents, multiple editions of most textbooks and monographs, including a significant number of titles pertinent to the subject in a recognized "standard" bibliography, an extensive collection of periodicals, including at least 65 percent of the titles pertinent to the subject which are included in *List of Journals Indexed in Index Medicus*. While English language materials may predominate, the collection usually contains important materials in French, German, Spanish, Russian and other languages. Older or superseded materials are usually retained for historical research.

Comprehensive level: A collection in which the library endeavors, insofar as possible, to include all significant works of recorded knowledge in all applicable languages for a defined and limited field. The scope of the collection and the level of collecting intensity are sufficiently broad to indicate a national resource for the subject. The aim, if not the achievement, is exhaustiveness.

EXAMPLE OF A GENERAL CRITERIA STATEMENT:

MEDICAL COLLEGE OF GEORGIA (AUGUSTA, GA)
GREENBLATT MEDICAL LIBRARY

General Criteria

A. Chronology - materials will be current, recently published materials.

B. Language - most materials will be in the English language.

C. Geography - most materials acquired will be national or international publications. The only local or regional items collected will be important state medical journals or will be published by or be about Georgia, Augusta, or the Medical College of Georgia.

D. Types of materials:

1. Dissertations - acquired very selectively, except all of those completed by students at MCG are collected.
2. Government documents - the MCG Library is a partial depository of health related government documents. Documents are acquired in accordance with the U.S. Government requirements.
3. Laboratory manuals - selectively acquired if they contain substantial explanatory content on procedures or techniques.
4. Foreign symposia or proceedings - only acquired through faculty request.
5. U.S. Symposia, proceedings - acquired through faculty request.
6. Examination questions, study guides - one in each core subject area is acquired if it is produced by a major scientific publisher.
7. Loose-leaf publications (updating services) - these are only acquired if they are important reference collection material or when other formats are not available.
8. Programmed texts - rarely acquired.
9. Reprints (collected journal articles) - not generally acquired.
10. Popular works - acquired very selectively for popular layman topics such as childbirth (see also leisure materials).
11. Consumer and patient education - rarely acquired except for AVs.
12. Transactions - are acquired in core subjects if they are timely.
13. Paperbacks - purchased if hardback is not available.
14. Newsletters, house organs - generally not acquired.
15. Catalogs - college, publisher, and AV producer catalogs are acquired.
16. Pamphlets and brochures - acquired for pamphlet file on both professional and layman level if free or of insignificant cost.
17. Leisure materials - small amount of journals for leisure reading, recommended by the Student Council, will be acquired; back issues will not be bound or kept.

18. Society bulletins - acquired only if they contain original research articles and/or substantive signed articles; state publications will be collected very selectively and generally ones primarily from this region.
19. Statistics - U.S. and Georgia health and vital statistics will be collected.
20. Current awareness services - not generally collected.
21. Abstracting journals - not generally collected.
22. Audiovisuals - generally, audiovisuals will be collected at the Support level (Level C) in the Core subjects (I). See separate policy.

E. Duplicates - only one copy of materials is acquired.

EXAMPLE OF A SERIALS SELECTION CRITERIA STATEMENT:

MASSACHUSETTS GENERAL HOSPITAL (BOSTON, MA)
TREADWELL MEDICAL LIBRARY

Selection Guidelines for Serials

1. Primary Responsibilities:

   The Director and the Assistant Director for Collection and Systems Management decide which titles are added to the collection, basing the decision on the following criteria.

2. Criteria for Selection:

   a. Titles requested by interlibrary loan at least five times per year over a period of four years, with six of these uses being for issues published in the most recent five years.
   b. Titles requested by members of the MGH Staff.
   c. Titles needed to support educational programs.
   d. Titles needed as the scope of the library expands or changes with new subspecialties or new programs in the institution.

3. Criteria for Retention:

   a. A title must be used at least six times per year as measured during journal use studies. When all journal volumes have been bar-coded, (by late 1991), the monitoring of journal use will be ongoing.
   b. Backfiles must show at least one use per year.

4. Serials Selection Procedures:

   a. Route user recommendations to the Assistant Director for Collection and Systems Management, who will send reply letter to user on decision or status of recommendation.
   b. Refer needs of new educational programs, new subspecialties or programs to the Director and Assistant Director for Collection and Systems Management.
   c. Report to the Director and Assistant Director for Collection and Systems Management results of annual journal use study listings:

      (1) Titles not meeting criteria.
      (2) Interlibrary loan titles meeting criteria for purchase.

   d. Assistant Director for Access Services sends for signature to the Assistant Director for Collection and Systems Management.

(1) New Journal Title Order Memo numbered sequentially and containing correct title, year and volume that the new subscription should begin with, and price.

(2) Journal Title Deletion Memo, numbered sequentially, containing title, price, and decision on retaining or discarding any or all volumes.

EXAMPLE OF A MONOGRAPHS SELECTION CRITERIA STATEMENT:

WASHINGTON UNIVERSITY (ST. LOUIS, MO)
MEDICAL LIBRARY

Monograph Evaluation Criteria

1. Bibliographic data: title, publisher, date, volumes, price.

2. Authority:
   > Is the author an M.D., Ph.D., or other specialist?
   > Has the author written any other books? Does the Library own them?
   > Is the author a recognized expert in the field?
   > Is the book relatively current? (Rarely is a book over 2 years old purchased, unless it is a replacement.)
   > Is the publisher reliable?
   > Has the publisher issued other sound titles?

3. Format:
   > Is the book easy to handle?
   > Is the binding durable?
   > Is the print easy on the eye?
   > Is the paper of good quality?
   > Are the illustrations reproduced well?

4. Bibliographic aids:
   > Is there a table of contents? Is it helpful?
   > Is there an index? Is it helpful?
   > Are there footnotes and bibliographies?
   > Are the charts, graphs, indexes helpful and clear?

5. Scope:
   > To what level is the book geared?
   > Is the coverage appropriate for the Library's collection?
   > Is the book technical, scholarly, or popular?

6. Aids in evaluation:
   > Is the book reviewed in journals? Are the reviews good or bad?
   > Is the book listed on the acquisitions lists of any other medical libraries?
   > Has the book been requested for purchase by a staff or faculty member?

EXAMPLES OF EXCERPTS FROM SUBJECT SECTIONS:

UNIVERSITY OF MICHIGAN (ANN ARBOR, MI)
ALFRED TAUBMAN MEDICAL LIBRARY

Gynecology (level 4):

Definition: A medical-surgical specialty concerned with the physiology and disorders of the female genital tract, as well as female endocrinology and reproductive physiology.

Level 4: Anatomy and physiology of female genital tract; pathology; medical and surgical treatment of gynecological disorders; contraception (see also birth control).

Hearing - see Audiology

Hematology (level 4):

Definition: Anatomy, physiology, pathology, symptomatology, and therapeutics related to blood and blood-forming tissues.

Level 4: Hemic and lymphatic systems and their diseases; bone marrow diseases; reticuloendothelial system.

Level 3: Blood banking - standards, management. Generally only materials related to practices in the U.S.

Histology (level 4):

Definition: Minute structure, composition, and function of tissues.

Level 4: Human histology; histochemistry; primate and laboratory animal histology.

Level 2: Representative works on comparative vertebrate histology. Some duplication with Natural Science Library.

History of medicine (level 3):

Level 4: History of nursing is collected quite comprehensively to support the research interests of the School of Nursing.

Level 3: Selected contemporary works on the history of medicine and related specialties, and pharmacy. Biographies of significant individuals, major institutions or associations, as well as more general works. All significant periodicals in the history of medicine are acquired.

Note: See section on Special Collections and Rare Books for collecting statement regarding special collections of primary materials. Some overlap with Graduate Library, particularly with medical biography and history of psychiatry.

UNIVERSITY OF CALIFORNIA, DAVIS (DAVIS, CA)
CARLSON HEALTH SCIENCES LIBRARY

Numbers in columns following the subject indicate ECS (Existing Collection Strength); and CC (Current Collecting Intensity)

Aerospace Medicine (NLM: WD700-758)	3F;3E
Allergy and Immunology (NLM: QW501-949)	3F;3E
History (HSL)	3F;3E
Hypersensitivity	4F;4E
Immunogenetics	4F; 4E
Immunologic Diseases (NLM: WD300-375)	4F;4E
Vaccines	4F;4E
Anatomy(NLM: Q51-102) (mostly at HSL)	4F;4E
Atlases	4F 3E
History (HSL)	3F;3E
Terminology	3F;3E
Comparative	4F;4E
Dissection	3F;3E
Anesthetic (NLM: WO200-460)	4F;4E
Anesthesia (mostly at HSL)	4E;4E
History (HSL)	3F;3E
Anesthetics	4F;4E
Ether	3E;3E
Hypnotism	3E;3E
Morphians	4E;4E
Neuromuscular Blocking Agents	4E;4E
Biochemistry (NLM: QU1-220)	4F;4E
Amino Acids	4F;4E
History (HSL)	3E;3E
Carbohydrates	3E;3E
Colloids	3E;3E
Enzymes	4F;4E
Hormones	4F;4E
Lipids	4F;4E

HOUSTON ACADEMY OF MEDICINE -TEXAS MEDICAL CENTER (HOUSTON, TX)
LIBRARY

NLM CLASS	SUBJECT	COLLECTION LEVEL
W	Medical economics	Instructional
	Manpower, distribution & characteristics	Instructional
	Medical practice management	Instructional
	Health services	Research
	Patient care	Research
	Medical social work	Basic
	Forensic medicine	Minimal
	medicolegal examination	Minimal
	medicolegal autopsy	Minimal
	suicide	Instructional
WA	PUBLIC HEALTH	
	Statistics	Basic
	History	Basic
	Social medicine	Basic
	Epidemiology	Research
	Biostatistics	Instructional
	theory & method	Instructional
	Preventive medicine	Instructional
	control & transmission of communicable diseases	Research
	Special groups	Basic
	maternal & child welfare	Instructional
	health in developing countries	Basic
	Occupational health	Minimal
	prevention & control	Minimal
	industrial accidents	Out of scope
	Health administration & organization	Instructional
	community health services	Instructional
	health education	Instructional
	Sanitation & environmental control	Out of scope
	water supply	Out of scope
	food additives	Minimal
	air sanitation	Out of scope
	waste disposal	Out of scope

NLM CLASS	SUBJECT	COLLECTION LEVEL

WB   PRACTICE OF MEDICINE

	Statistics	Basic
	Directories	Basic
	US & Texas	Research
	Education	Instructional
	computer-assisted instruction	Basic
	History	Research
	Medical practice	Research
	Family practice	Research

EXAMPLES OF EXCERPTS FROM FORMATS SECTIONS:

NATIONAL INSTITUTES OF HEALTH (BETHESDA, MD)
LIBRARY

— DISSERTATIONS & THESES —These are rarely collected.
— EDITIONS —New editions of works already owned are collected in relation to use of previous editions.
— ENCYCLOPEDIAS — Major general and special subject English language encyclopedias are collected. Superseded and older editions are retained for reference purposes, when appropriate.
— EXAMINATION GUIDES — Examination guides intended for medical students and physicians are collected very selectively.
— FACT SHEETS — These are not collected unless they contain substantive data related to NIH.
— FICTION — Fictional and other literary works, including those written by or about medical professionals and the medical community are not collected.
— GOVERNMENT PUBLICATIONS — Federal publications with emphasis on scientific and medical research, education and legislation are collected selectively. Legislative documents (U.S. public laws, legislative histories, proposed legislation, etc.) with emphasis on biomedical and Department of Health and Human Services issues are collected selectively.
— JOURNALS — Major journals covering subjects relating to the NIH research activities are collected comprehensively. Peripheral subjects are collected very selectively in English only. Journals of societies, hospitals, and other organizations are collected only if they contain original research results or substantive signed articles. Those containing only social news or simplified discussions of medical procedures are not collected.
—LOOSE-LEAF PUBLICATIONS — Publications periodically updated by replacement pages are collected only if essential.
— MANUALS — Laboratory manuals are rarely collected. Workbooks (providing questions and answers) are not collected.
— MICROFORMS — Microform versions of journals are collected if a hard copy is unavailable, or if the micro format would provide a more cost-effective method of acquisition or would conserve space.

UNIVERSITY OF MICHIGAN (ANN ARBOR, MI)
ALFRED TAUBMAN MEDICAL LIBRARY

Dissertations
Masters theses from the U.M. School of Nursing and dissertations from the College of Pharmacy, School of Nursing, and Medical School (through Rackham) are collected. The library has fairly complete holdings for nursing and pharmacy.

Dissertations and theses from other institutions are not purchased. If a non-U.M. dissertation is requested and is unavailable through interlibrary loan, the requester is given information for ordering a personal copy.

Electronic publications

Databases, texts, journals and other information files available in electronic format are accessible (for a fee) when offered by standard database vendors. Both self-service and librarian-mediated searching is available. At present the library does not provide direct access to locally produced or purchased electronic publications or files.

Examination review books; study guides

Books that are intended to help students or foreign medical graduates prepare for National Board or specialty examinations are rarely purchased. A very few of those most heavily requested and issued by a major medical publisher or professional organization may be acquired. Outdated editions should be withdrawn.

Fiction

Fictional works written by physicians or other health professionals are not acquired by the library. The are considered literature and when appropriate would be acquired by the Graduate Library. Likewise, fiction written about physicians or using a medical setting are excluded from the collection.

Government documents

The University of Michigan is a partial depository library for U.S. government publications. The major holdings are in the Documents Center. The majority of depository documents issued by the Department of Health and Human Services and its subdivisions are housed at the Public Health Library, and those emanating from the National Library of Medicine are at the Taubman Medical Library. Except for a few important medical serials, occasional reports of major importance, and publications acquired for reference use, Taubman collects very few government documents.

EXAMPLE OF A SPECIAL POLICY STATEMENT ON GIFTS AND DUPLICATES:

WASHINGTON UNIVERSITY (ST. LOUIS, MO)
MEDICAL LIBRARY

Gifts

While the Medical Library appreciates gifts of print and nonprint materials that are in scope as defined in this Manual, it reserves the right to refuse, add, exchange, sell, or discard gift materials as it sees fit. The Library does not evaluate gifts monetarily, but does acknowledge them by letter or acknowledgment form.

Duplicates

Monographs - Duplicate copies of monographs are collected only if a title on course reserve is used so heavily that purchase of an additional copy for course reserve or circulation is warranted, or additional copies of a title are necessary for Library staff use.

Serials - Second copies of titles are not purchased with the exception of bibliographic tools used by the Library staff. Second copies of Main Reading Room titles that are received as gifts on a regular basis from an established source and are approved by the Reference staff are retained for a limited period of time. Second copies of titles shelved in other locations that are received as gifts are not retained.

EXAMPLE OF A SPECIAL POLICY STATEMENT ON MULTIPLE COPIES AND REPLACEMENTS:

THOMAS JEFFERSON UNIVERSITY (PHILADELPHIA, PA)
SCOTT MEMORIAL LIBRARY

Multiple Copies

Books - Duplication of monographic materials is limited to those titles with a demonstrated exceptionally high demand, usually textbooks and other titles kept in the Reserve collection to support specific course work. Duplicate copies are weeded when heavy demand ceases. Dictionaries, manuals and Brandon-Hill monographs are duplicated when copies are useful in more than one location, e.g., Reference, Reserve, Basic Reading Room. A copy of all current health sciences books acquired for the Jeffersoniana Collection is also added to the circulating book collection.

Journals - Multiple subscriptions to journals are entered for titles in the Basic Reading Room which are retained for three years and are not bound and for a select few other titles which are heavily used, (e.g. some of the Saunders' clinics series).

Learning Resource Center - Audiovisual material that is in constant demand is collected in duplicate. Duplicate copies of microcomputer software packages are purchased in accordance with copyright restrictions and need. Legitimate copies of software are purchased for each workstation. The volume of usage and price are factors in determining the number of copies which are supported. A license agreement for duplication of heavily used software packages will be purchased whenever possible.

Replacements

Books - Missing titles from the general monograph, Reference, PERC, Basic Reading Room and Reserve collections are not automatically replaced. The decision is made by the Collection Development Librarian and is based on subject matter, currentness, usage, price and budget restraints; new editions are always preferred if available. Books missing from the Browsing Room collection are not replaced.

Journals - Missing journal issues or volumes are replaced whenever possible to prevent gaps in the Library's holdings. Issues from second copies may be used to complete copy one holdings for binding. No attempt is made to replace missing issues for the Browsing Room journals.

EXAMPLE OF A SPECIAL POLICY STATEMENT ON RETENTION:

UNIVERSITY OF ARIZONA (TUCSON, AZ)
ARIZONA HEALTH SCIENCES LIBRARY

Retention
Following are general guidelines for retention of materials:

1. Special Collections
   The Library has assumed an archival responsibility for materials in Special Collections. These materials are not weeded.

2. General Collection
   This collection, for the most part, is retained indefinitely.

3. Reference Collection
   Subject histories, textbooks, biographies, dictionaries, and encyclopedias may be weeded if they are more than ten years old, and if more current material sufficient to meet the Library's needs has been added to the collection.

Major journals, abstracting and indexing services and major subject bibliographies are retained indefinitely in whatever format is judged most convenient.

Other reference titles which are serial in nature and which have material which is updated and/or superseded are treated in one of two ways:

   1. Latest at reference. Materials which could have an extended use beyond that of the current edition.

   2. Latest only in library. Titles whose content is totally superseded by that of the next edition. These sorts of titles are withdrawn from the AHS Library upon receipt and processing of the newest edition.

EXAMPLE OF A SPECIAL POLICY STATEMENT ON PRESERVATION:

UNIVERSITY OF MICHIGAN (ANN ARBOR, MI)
ALFRED TAUBMAN MEDICAL LIBRARY

XI. Preservation

A. Environment

The proper environment for preserving the collections should be maintained. Temperature and humidity should be kept within the ranges recommended by the University Library Preservation Office and fluctuations minimized as much as possible. Levels should be monitored as necessary and problems addressed.

Housekeeping standards should be maintained in order to prevent and eliminate insects or the accumulation of dust on the collections.

Rare books and special collections should be housed in an environment that affords a constant environment with optimal levels of temperature, humidity, and light, as well as proper shelving and protection from theft.

B. Physical Care

All staff who work with library materials should be taught how to handle them properly. Those who supervise or train shelving, photocopy, bindery preparation, or interlibrary loan staff, or others who handle materials frequently should take advantage of workshops held by the Preservation Office.

All staff should be encouraged to identify and report volumes needing repair or replacement.
Whenever possible books and journals should be shelved upright (or flat, if very large) with proper support. Sufficient room should be left on each shelf so volumes may be removed easily without pulling on the spine.

Facilities for returning materials after use should be provided conveniently - by the circulation desk, photocopiers, and in the stacks. When possible, use of book returns should be avoided. If used, they should be designed to minimize damage, and should be emptied frequently. Materials moved on trucks within the library or transported to sites outside the library should be handled to prevent damage.

C. Collection Management

Binding specifications for journals should be selected for maximum long-term preservation - to withstand use as well as to conserve the paper. Titles of permanent value should be bound as soon as possible. Ideally, journals should be bound when all issues in a volume have been received (or the number that will constitute a bound volume). Paper books to be bound should receive binding on receipt whenever practical. Books that have sturdy paper bindings and anticipated low use may not be bound until the need is evident. Books not considered to be of permanent value - multiple copies, reserve materials not generally within scope, etc. - may never be bound.

Decisions about worn, damaged, or deteriorating materials will depend on judgment of their permanent research value as well as their physical state and the options for preservation. Replacement, withdrawal, rebinding, repair, or other conservation measures may all be considered. Choices should be consistent with the general collection development policy. Local repairs should be made with materials that have the least potential for causing future damage and should follow guidelines developed by the Preservation Office. Staff who undertake minor repairs should receive proper training. Questions about restoration or major conservation treatment for valuable items, should be referred to the Preservation Office for advice.

D. Emergencies and Disasters

The library should be prepared for minor emergencies, such as ceiling leaks. Plastic sheeting should be kept available and staff should know where to locate it.

The library should also have a plan for handling major disasters, such as fire or water, so that immediate action can be taken to protect or conserve the collections.

EXAMPLE OF A SPECIAL POLICY STATEMENT ON WITHDRAWAL:

MEDICAL UNIVERSITY OF SOUTH CAROLINA (CHARLESTON, SC)
MEDICAL LIBRARY

Guidelines for Withdrawal of Materials

Weeding the library's collection is part of the evaluating process and is an on-going process. Outdated or inappropriate materials, which are not of historical importance, will be withdrawn. The following guidelines are built into the Library's normal procedures and routines.

1. Only the latest edition of non-medical reference works such as almanacs, Europa Yearbook, biographical or organizational directories, etc., are kept.
2. Directories of medical organizations which include biographical information such as the AMA American Medical Directory, or the Directory of Medical Specialists are kept.
3. Newsletters and other miscellaneous materials of ephemeral interest are kept for one year.
4. Materials in poor condition are removed from the collection and either replaced, repaired or withdrawn according to the usefulness of the item.

A comprehensive weeding should be done every five years.

The Collection Development Librarian with the help of the Collection Development Committee has responsibility for weeding activities. The following guidelines are to be used in evaluating each item:

1. Books not checked out in the last ten years are pulled for further evaluation.
2. Out-of-scope material no longer relevant to the needs of the university are removed.
3. Duplicate copies of texts ten years or older are withdrawn.
4. Duplicate copies of serials not used heavily are withdrawn whereas back-files of duplicate copies of journals of high use are kept for fifteen years.
5. All materials known to be of historical importance are retained.
6. One copy of each edition of standard or "classic" texts such as *Harrison's Principles of Medicine* or *William's Obstetrics* are kept. Other texts published in numerous editions are weeded selectively. The first edition and representative later editions at approximately ten years ' interval are generally kept.
7. In general, serials indexed by standard indexing and abstracting services are kept.

All books not circulated within the last ten years will be checked against Garrison and Morton for their historical importance before they are withdrawn permanently from the collection.

EXAMPLES OF HOSPITAL LIBRARY COLLECTION DEVELOPMENT POLICIES:

MAINE MEDICAL CENTER (PORTLAND, ME)
LIBRARY

Collection Development Policy

Purpose:

This document has been developed as a guide to assist the Library in the exercising of its collection development responsibilities. The immense number of materials available and increased book, serial and audio-visual material prices and increased processing costs make it mandatory that the Library have a written collection development policy which stresses wise selection to strengthen the resources of the Library. Such a document necessarily cannot be definitive for all time. The Library is not a rigidly fixed entity but a constantly changing and evolving institution, mirroring the needs of the Maine Medical Center.

The Library must be informed of forthcoming research and the development of new services and programs as a certain lead time is necessary to acquire materials to support these programs. The objective of the collection development policy must reflect the long range goals of the Medial Center. Any collection building in weak areas must proceed at a gradual rate without neglecting the strengths of the collection. If large scale building of these weak areas is indicated, additional funding from the Medical Center is necessary.

The collection development policy must also take into consideration the fact that the library cannot be self-sufficient. Publishing output has reached such proportions that no one Library can obtain all materials needed. Libraries depend on interlibrary loan systems for borrowing infrequently used materials that are not locally available.

Collection Development Objectives:

The Library's primary function is to provide the necessary informational resources to support the Medical Center's basic responsibilities of patient care, teaching, research, continuing education and administration. To meet this obligation, the development of the Library's collections should largely reflect the current and long-range emphasis and commitment placed on these responsibilities and on the individual programs supporting them by the Medical Center. Those charged with the development of the collection must consider a variety of factors including the level of patient care, education and research programs within the institution, the rate of publication, the cost of materials in various disciplines, and the dependency of the various disciplines on library support. Special attention will be given to the support of new programs.

The primary collection development objective is to provide those books; serials; pamphlets; audio-visual materials; archives; databases and other information sources needed in support of the Medical Center's basic responsibilities as a teaching and clinical care institution.

Selection responsibility:

All librarians are responsible for taking an active role in suggesting or initiating purchases. Each purchase should be made within the framework of this document. The selection process involves the following factors:

1. Judging the completeness of holdings.
2. Determining the relative importance of all formats of materials for each discipline.
3. Encouraging hospital employees to participate in selection by suggesting new titles.
4. Studying use patterns (circulation statistics, etc.) to determine areas of great demand or areas in which the collection is not well represented.

Final authority for selection rests with the Director of Library Services and those to whom she/he delegates such authority. However, the Director assumes legal responsibility.

Levels of collection intensity:

The Library's depth of collection in each subject field reflects the demands made by students, medical staff and employees. The following levels are those towards which the Library strives:

Research level:
A collection which includes the major source materials required for independent research, including materials containing research reporting, scientific experimental results and other information useful to researchers. It includes all monographs; a very extensive collection of journals and major materials are retained for historical research. NOTE: At present the MMC Library is not purchasing at this level. As research efforts gain greater momentum within the Medical Center, certain areas will be reviewed for material to support these research efforts.

Support level:
A collection which is adequate to maintain knowledge of a subject required for limited or generalized purposes, of less than research intensity. It includes a wide range of basic monographs; a selection of representative journals and the reference tools and fundamental bibliographical sources pertaining to the subject.

Basic level:
> A highly selective collection which serves to introduce and define the subject, and to indicate the varieties of information available elsewhere. Such a collection includes major dictionaries and encyclopedias; selected editions of important works; general surveys; important bibliographies and a few major periodicals in the field. A basic information collection is not sufficiently intensive to support independent study in the subject area involved. It may include strong retrospective holdings in discontinued areas of former interest to the Library and/or material selected for its relevance to other areas of strength.

Survey level:
> A subject area which is out of scope for the Library, in which few selections are made beyond reference works. The collection contains only a few major items which take a broad look at the clinical aspects of the subject.

B	Philosophy, Psychology, Religion	Survey
E	History, America	Survey
G	Geography, Anthropology, Recreation	Survey
H	Social Sciences	Survey
K	Law	Survey
L	Education	Survey
P	Language & Literature	Survey
Q	Science	Survey
QA	Mathematics	Survey
QC	Physics	Survey
QD	Chemistry	Survey
QH	Natural History	Survey
QS	Human Anatomy	Basic
QT	Physiology	Basic
QU	Biochemistry	Support
QV	Pharmacology	Support
QW	Microbiology & Immunology	Basic
QX	Parasitology	Basic
QY	Clinical Pathology	Support
QZ	Pathology	Support
W	Medical Profession	Support
WA	Public Health	Support
WB	Practice of Medicine	Support
WC	Infectious Disease	Basic
WD 100	Deficiency Disease	Basic
WD 200	Metabolic Disease	Basic
WD 300	Diseases of Allergy	Basic
WD 400	Animal Poisoning	Basic
WD 500	Plant Poisoning	Survey

WD 600	Diseases caused by Physical Agents	Basic
WD 700	Aviation and Space Medicine	Basic
WE	Musculoskeletal System	Support
WF	Respiratory System	Support
WG	Cardiovascular System	Support
WH	Hemic and Lymphatic Systems	Basic
WI	Gastrointestinal System	Support
WJ	Urogenital System	Support
WK	Endocrine System	Support
WL	Nervous System	Support
WM	Psychiatry	Support
WN	Radiology	Basic
WO	Surgery	Support
WP	Gynecology	Support
WQ	Obstetrics	Support
WR	Dermatology	Basic
WS	Pediatrics	Support
WT	Geriatrics, Chronic Disease	Basic
WU	Dentistry, Oral Surgery	Survey
WV	Otorhinolaryngology	Basic
WW	Ophthalmology	Basic
WX	Hospitals	Support
WY	Nursing	Support
WZ	History of Medicine	Basic

Selection Criteria:

General Criteria for Selection of Library Materials:
The following criteria are to be observed by librarians in the selection of any materials, whether monograph, serial or audio-visual, for the Library collection:

1. The importance of the subject matter to the collection.
2. Timeliness or permanence of the material.
3. Authoritativeness.
4. Accuracy of information.
5. The technical excellence, durability and readability of the format.
6. The author's reputation and credibility in the field.
7. Inclusion of the title in recognized bibliographies.
8. Price.
9. Availability of materials on the subject.

Criteria for selecting monographs:

A monograph is a single volume, dealing systematically and in detail with one subject or class of subjects. This definition includes monographic series and reference sources such as encyclopedias, almanacs and biographical sources. Monographs are selected for the Library's collection primarily to serve the clinical needs of the Medical Center community.

In addition to the General Criteria the following criteria will be weighed in the selection of books for the Library's collection:

1. Possible positive review evaluation in one or more of the accepted reviewing media/or citations of the materials in specialized bibliographies or indexes.
2. Reputation of the publisher.
3. If the price is over $75.00, a local "expert" in that field will be consulted.
4. Only English language books will be purchased, except in the case of foreign language dictionaries.
5. Materials necessary for interlibrary loan, verification, selection and other support function.
6. Title written by Medical Center personnel.
7. Book completes series holdings.
8. Whether book is a new edition with revised information or merely a reprint.
9. For illustrated volumes either reputation of illustrator or quality of reproduction.

Criteria for the Selection of Serials:

Serial subscriptions for the Library are selected to cover, as broad as possible, all fields relating to the clinical and educational goals of the hospital, while also supplying specific and deep coverage in fields where the need is indicated.

New serial titles will be considered for purchase when a department or the Library is willing to drop titles that are no longer relevant. If the decision is made to order a serial, the intention is to retain it as a permanent part of the collection in as complete a run as possible.

Most of the future additions to the retrospective collection shall be microfiche or other format which condenses the space utilized for the collection. This will include annual volumes of many of the periodicals and journals which have formerly been bound. The paper volumes will be kept for a varying length of time.

Depending on the availability of funds, complete runs of as many journals as possible will be replaced by microfilm. Those journals with the first priority for replacement in microfilm will be those which are used most and which are stolen or mutilated most. In the future, some journals which must be retained in the collection, but are rarely used, will be purchased only in microform.

Serial selection and evaluation is made by the Public Services, Technical Services/Media Services librarians, working in conjunction with the Director of Library Services. The Librarians are responsible for keeping the serials collection in balance, weighing the programs offered, the educational and research activities. Further, the Librarians are responsible for determining which journal titles will be listed in the various networks in which the Library participates.

All serials are subject to re-evaluation on an annual basis. The following criteria, in addition to the General Criteria for Selection are to be weighed in the selection of any serial title:

1. Evaluation should be based on a sample copy and/or a table of contents with a photocopy of three randomly selected articles and/or a review.
2. The journal is indexed or abstracted by services available in the Library.
3. Accuracy and relative objectivity of the content.
4. Frequency with which serial is cited in the literature.
5. Only English language titles are purchased.
6. Consideration of the necessity of duplicating any title available in departmental libraries.
7. A decision to acquire a new serial title must take into account the holdings of other libraries in the local area.
8. Serials necessary for interlibrary loan verification.
9. For serials not indexed or abstracted serious consideration must be given to the timeliness of the subject.
10. Consideration should be given to potential for usage.
11. When a title is recommended for addition to the collection, a review of the current subscription in that field should be conducted.
12. When a new subscription is approved, consideration should be given to purchasing a two-year back run in the least expensive format.
13. To support a new program a minimal two to three-year back run of a serial title should be purchased in the least expensive format.
14. Any serial subject to a significant increase in cost must be re-evaluated.
15. In the case of annuals, serious consideration should be given to buying the titles every second or third year.
16. Serials will not be purchased solely to support one individual's research.
17. No serial will be purchased for the display and discard shelf.

Criteria for selecting audio-visuals:

Non-print media is gaining recognition equal to that of printed materials. As with the selection of monographs one seeks the best material available in terms of effectiveness, authority, currency, etc. Because the quality of the technical aspects of any audio-visual directly relates to the effectiveness of its use, audio-visual material will be ordered on a preview basis and evaluated before a final determination of purchase is made. Final authority on the technical quality will rest with the Library Media Center staff and the final authority on the purchase will rest with the Director of Library Services.

The high cost of non-print media, even though evaluated as excellent, imposes limitation on their purchase. The selection of audio-visuals, although based on the same principles as the selection of books, must also take into consideration the technical aspects (quality of photography, sound track, narration, etc.) of the product. The following criteria represent the general criteria to be considered in the selection of audio-visuals:

1. Content of material must be in direct clinical support or a potential for use in more than one department can be demonstrated.
2. Subject content, treatment and presentation must be on an appropriate level; patient education materials will not be purchased routinely.
3. Reputation of the producer.
4. Technical quality of color, sound, continuity, etc.
5. Currency and timeliness of the material. Rapidly changing subjects should be purchased in less expensive media.
6. Cost effectiveness of one media over another, or over the printed word.
7. Whether preview or other adequate review process is provided.
8. Weakness of the collection in a particular subject area.
9. Projected images must be sufficiently large and bright.
10. English language productions only will be purchased.
11. Durability of the physical item.
12. Appropriateness of selected audio-visual format for use in a subject field.
13. Commercialism to be held to an acceptable level, not distracting from the central theme and content.
14. There is commitment to continued use of the media.

Multiple copies:

In order to provide the broadest possible range of materials in support of the Medical Center's programs, the Library will not normally purchase multiple copies of books, serials, or audio-visuals. Requests for multiple copies will be considered individually according to present needs and the value of the resource as part of the Library's permanent collection. In the instances where a decision is made to purchase multiple copies, the additional copies will be acquired in the most economical format.

Replacements:

Resources that are lost, missing or withdrawn because of wear will not automatically be replaced. The merit of the book, serial, or audio-visual must be considered by the Director before replacement copies are authorized. Demand for the resource, its value to the collection and whether or not it has been superseded by a new edition or newer material should be considered as criteria in requesting replacements.

Out-of-print materials:

The Library will not try to replace or purchase out-of-print materials. However, if such materials can be located as a gift to the Library and are deemed important to the collection, they will be gratefully received.

Commercially sponsored materials:

Commercially or privately sponsored books, pamphlets, and audio-visual materials will be acceptable for the Library if they fulfill the following criteria:

1. The materials supplement or enrich the collection.
2. The materials meet the same standards for selection as applied to purchases.
3. The amount of corporate advertising is kept to a minimum and is tastefully presented.

Databases:

The Library currently contracts for access to a large number of computer searchable bibliographic databases. These services are used to provide subject searching and bibliographic data retrieval to employees. The subjects covered by these databases are wide-ranging. The databases and their corresponding vendors are chosen in order to provide useful and appropriate coverage for the support of the Medical Center's programs.

The Library will continue to evaluate this database selection in order to keep it closely aligned with the hospital's mission. Furthermore, the Library will begin to explore the relationship of these databases to print indexes and abstracts. Studies will be undertaken to determine whether current databases can be used to replace expensive print sources.

Gifts:

The Library will accept donations of books and other publications as well as gifts of money designated for the purchase of library materials, in accordance with the following criteria:

1. Potential donors should be requested to provide in advance a list of materials being offered so that their value to the collection may be assessed. In cases where the gift involves five or less titles, they may be checked over the telephone without a list.
2. Publications received in the Library as gifts will be reviewed by the same standards as applied to new materials being selected.
3. Gift materials must be of such a nature that they can be integrated into the collection and not require special facilities, control, or staffing.
4. Gift materials requiring continuing obligations on the part of the Library should not be accepted without serious consideration of the Library's ability to keep the material up-to-date.
5. Normally, the Library will not accept added copies of materials already in the collection.
6. The value of the gift should be weighed against space limitations and the cost of processing the materials.
7. The Library has the right to retain or dispose of any gift materials at the discretion of the librarians. Donors should be made aware of this and items 1-6.
8. The policy regarding the acceptance of gift periodicals (back issues of journals, whether long runs or scattered issues) is to decline the gift unless the issue or issues fill a gap in the collection. The exception should be the offer of a rare or costly set which the Library does not have. An individual decision would have to be made by the Director for each offer.
9. The Library will abide by the regulations of gifts as outlined in the "Statement of Appraisal of Gifts" developed by the Committee on Manuscript Collections of the Association of College and Research Libraries which is stated as follows:

   1. The appraisal of a gift to a library for tax purposes generally is the responsibility of the donor since it is the donor who benefits from the tax deduction. Generally, the cost of the appraisal should be borne by the donor.
   2. The library should at all times protect the interests of its donors as best it can and should suggest the desirability of appraisals whenever such a suggestion would be in order.
   3. To protect both its donors and itself, the library as an interested party, ordinarily should not appraise gifts made to it. It is recognized, however, that on occasion the library may wish to appraise small gifts, since many of them are not worth the time and expense an outside appraisal requires. Generally, however, the library will limit its assistance to the donor to:

    a. providing her/him with information such as dealers' catalogs;
    b. suggestions of appropriate professional appraisers who might be consulted;
    c. administrative and processing services which would assist the appraiser in making an accurate evaluation.

4. The acceptance of a gift which has been appraised by a third, and disinterested party, does not in any way imply an endorsement of the appraisal by the library.
5. An archivist, curator, or librarian, if he/she is conscious that as an expert he/she may have to prove his competence in court, may properly act as an independent appraiser of library materials. He/She should not in any way suggest that his/her appraisal is endorsed by his/her library (such as by the use of the library's letterhead), nor should he/she ordinarily act in this fashion (except when handling small gifts) if his/her institution is to receive the donation.

Gift Policy written July 30, 1982;
Reviewed February, 1987;
Reviewed December 1989

Weeding:

Weeding involves the removal of materials from the active collection for discarding or transferring to the historical collection. the purpose of weeding is to re-evaluate the collection in conjunction with the selection of new and replacement materials. An active and continuous weeding program is essential in order to keep the collection viable and useful. Primary responsibility for weeding the collection rests with the Librarians. the following guidelines will be followed:

1. Weeding will not be done solely on the basis of circulation statistics or past use, although these will be considered.
2. A work containing outdated or inaccurate information, if it is not valuable for historical or research purposes, should be discarded.
3. An irreparably deteriorated, mutilated or damaged work should be weeded. If a replacement is unavailable for an item still needed in the collection, every effort should be made to preserve it.
4. Weeding should not tend to bias the collections.
5. Serials duplicated by microforms in the collection should be considered for weeding.
6. Superseded editions should be considered for retention, depending on subject matter, length of time between editions, circulation, and extent of revisions.

Materials selected for discarding will be disposed of through give-away shelves, exchange, or simply through the Medical Center's trash mechanism. All property stamps will be covered with a withdrawn stamp.

The process of weeding a collection is of equal importance to the original selection of materials. They are in fact two sides of one coin representing the maintenance of a vital, useful, well-kept collection. As in the selection process, the recommendations and assistance of Medical Center staff are essential and will be given full consideration. The final decision will rest with the Director of Library Services in case of disputed items.

ST. JOSEPH HOSPITAL (ORANGE, CA) BURLEW MEDICAL LIBRARY

I. Authority Establishing the Policy:
  A. The selection policy of the Burlew Medical Library shall be agreed upon by:
    (1) The Medical Librarian;
    (2) Assistant Administrator to whom Medical Librarian reports;
    (3) Library Committee.

II. Purpose:
The selection policy of the Burlew Medical Library serves as a guide to the selection of books, documents, journals, and audiovisual materials which contribute to the clinical, educational, and research activities of both St. Joseph Hospital and Children's Hospital of Orange County.

III. Scope Statement:
  A. The scope of the Burlew Medical Library's Collection shall consist of books, documents, journals, and audiovisual materials which will aid in meeting the clinical and education information needs, and to a lesser extent, the research needs of the Staff and Employees of St. Joseph Hospital and Children's Hospital of Orange County.

  B. The Selection Policy recognizes a firm commitment to collect informational materials at the physician level, as well as at the nursing, technician, and support staff level. The library will not commit to collecting informational materials at the nursing student or resident level.

    (1) The Burlew Medical Library recognizes the patient's right to understand his/her illness/health situation in lay terms and, as funds are available, will collect at the lay level.

  C. Foreign language books will be purchased only if the equivalent information is not available in an English language publication.

  D. The library does not commit to providing a collection of historical materials; rather, the library commits to the first and second priorities of informational materials that contribute to patient care and in service/continuing education needs. If, however, the library receives gifts of a historical nature, these gifts as deemed appropriate by the Medical Librarian and as time permits, will be added to the library's historical collection.

COLUMBIA HOSPITAL (MILWAUKEE, WI)
MEDICAL LIBRARY

Purpose:
This policy provides guidelines for building and maintaining a collection of information resources adequate for the current needs of hospital staff. In general, the most up-to-date, authoritative materials directly pertinent to patient care, education and administrative programs and activities will be purchased. Judgment as to whether specific materials meet these criteria is exercised by the library staff in conjunction with physicians, managers, and other health professionals. Every effort will be made to purchase the best sources available within the financial limits of the Library's annual budget.

Scope and Coverage:
The SCOPE of the collection refers to the range of its subject content. COVERAGE refers to the depth or penetration into a subject area. Coverage within the Medical Library collection is at the "skeletal" or "reference" level depending on the needs of primary clientele working in a particular field or program area, defined as follows:

"skeletal" - includes the latest editions of one or two texts and bibliographic access through indexes and databases.

"reference" - includes skeletal coverage plus additional texts and reference books, one or more journals, and retrospective sources as appropriate.

For each profession and occupational group represented in the Hospital, the Library will provide, at the minimum, current materials at the "skeletal" level. Those subjects for which the Library attempts to provide "reference" coverage include:

Allergy & Immunology	Nursing
Anesthesiology	Nutrition
Cardiovascular Diseases	Obstetrics & Gynecology
Critical Care Medicine	Occupational Medicine
Dermatology	Oncology
Diabetes	Ophthalmology
Emergency Medicine	Orthopedics
Endocrinology	Otolaryngology
Family Medicine	Pathology
Gastroenterology	Pharmacology
Geriatric Psychiatry	Physical Medicine
Health Administration	Psychiatry
Health Education	Radiology
Hematology	Rehabilitation
Infectious Diseases	Respiratory Diseases
Laboratory Medicine	Rheumatic Diseases
Management	Sports Medicine

Medical Profession	Surgery
Neurology	Urology

The Medical Library does not attempt to cover any subject at the "research" level, i.e. coverage that would permit independent clinical research. Nor does the Library select materials in any languages other than English.

The scope of the Library's collections falls primarily within the fields of clinical medicine, pre-clinical sciences, nursing, allied health, and management topics that apply to professionals working in the Hospital. Literature in most fields may be considered for acquisition if a reasonable portion of the material is relevant to the needs of the Library's user groups. In addition, reference tools necessary for internal library operations will be acquired.

Criteria for Selection:
When selecting books or audiovisuals, the following criteria will be considered:

- Authority (author, date, publisher/producer)
- Quality (readability or audibility)
- Bibliographic aids (indexes, references, graphs)
- Subject scope and coverage (suitable for intended audience)
- Extent to which subject is covered by current subscriptions.
- Outside evaluation (reviews, requests from users)
- Price

When selecting journals, the following criteria will be considered:

- Authority (publisher/editorial board, journal referred)
- Indexed in major indexes or databases
- Subject scope and coverage (suitable for intended audience)
- Extent to which subject is covered by current subscriptions
- Usage (requested 5 times or more on interlibrary loan)
- Price

Audiovisuals:
Selection of audiovisual materials will follow the same scope and coverage criteria as printed materials. The Library currently purchases materials in only two formats: audiocassettes and VHS videocassettes.

Special Collections:
Patient/Consumer Collection

A small collection of non-technical books, pamphlets, periodicals, and videocassettes is maintained in the Library to meet the needs of patients, their families and the general public. Selection is based on subject needs as expressed by patients and consumers, using the criteria outlined for the selection of professional materials.

Management Collection:

For individuals interested in the business of health care, the Library maintains a collection of books and periodicals on health care administration, human resource development, customer service, financial management, and other general management topics. Selection is based on the same criteria as for other professional materials.

Department Collection:

Holdings of books and journals in departmental libraries will be limited to frequently used materials and will be paid for by the individual department. Books will be cataloged by the library staff at the request of the department and incorporated into the Library's card catalog. The library staff will periodically inventory the journal holdings of other departments and incorporate these records into the hospital-wide journal holdings list published by the Library.

Gifts:

Gifts are accepted with the understanding that the library may use the material as needs dictate. This means that donated items may be integrated into the collection, used for exchange with other libraries, or discarded. Gifts will be acknowledged in writing by the Director of Library Services. No evaluation of gifts for tax purposes will be made by library staff. Donors are encouraged to contact the IRS for information regarding deductions applicable to their gifts.

Replacements:

Current books that are lost will be evaluated on an individual basis to determine the necessity for replacement. Book replacement decisions will be based on the following criteria:

- Age of material;
- Probability of a new edition within the next year; and
- Usage data.

When current journals are lost, the library staff will seek to replace them through journal exchange with other libraries as soon as possible. For key titles, a decision may be made to purchase a replacement copy.

NEWTON-WELLESLEY HOSPITAL (NEWTON, MA)
LIBRARY

I. Collection Development:

A regular program of selection, acquisition and weeding shall keep the collection current and relevant. Materials in all forms shall be considered for the collection. The scope of the collection shall be broad, to directly support the information needs of the entire hospital community. Priority, however, will be given to those clinical materials required by the medical staff, nursing service, medical-teaching and ancillary-teaching programs which impact directly on patient care decision making. Selection and retention of materials shall be coordinated with other cooperating libraries in order to broaden availability and prevent unnecessary duplication.

All Library users may recommend materials to be purchased for the collection. Recommendations are reviewed by the Library Director who makes the final selection using the guidance of the Library Committee and subject specialists, as well as the following criteria:

- Standard lists (recommendations of necessary books in hospital libraries).
- Subject scope (related to program activity within the Hospital).
- Current coverage of the subject by materials already in the collection.
- Availability of the item elsewhere in the Hospital or through interlibrary loan.
- Reputation of the author or publisher.
- Cost.
- Timeliness (generally books no more than three years old will be purchased).
- Technical quality of the publication.
- Review by subject experts.

Those materials selected may be purchased through one of the following funds:

- Hospital Budget (general materials).
- Medical Staff Dues (Clinical Reserve materials and medical/surgical journal binding).
- Stellar Fund (materials relating to diabetes and endocrinology).
- Stearns/West Fund (Clinical Reserve materials).
- Bertha Allen Library (Nursing materials).

Gifts shall be received with appreciation, but will not be subject to any restrictions. Large gifts may not necessarily be retained or housed together. Gifts which are retained will be acknowledged, but will not be appraised for monetary value. Gifts are not automatically accepted but must be reviewed for suitability by the Library Director.

The collection will be reviewed regularly to eliminate those materials which are out of date, no longer used, and are of no historical value. Materials which are to be withdrawn will be reviewed by subject experts before being discarded. Withdrawals will be disposed of by sale, exchange or discard.

Signed by Executive Vice President and Chief Operating Officer

LONG BEACH COMMUNITY HOSPITAL (LONG BEACH, CA) LIBRARY

Policy:

This library shall maintain a collection of books, journals, and audiovisuals designed to meet the informational, educational, and research-related needs of the medical and hospital staffs.

Level of Coverage:

Broad, general coverage will be provided for each professional and occupational group on the medical and hospital staff. Specialized materials will be provided on a comprehensive level in the fields of internal medicine, cardiology, oncology, surgery, geriatrics, nursing, and hospital administration. As the hospital needs change this level of coverage will change. Materials on a basic level only will be provided in the basic sciences. Foreign language publications will not be collected.

Currency of the Collection:

New editions of the basic books and texts shall be acquired as published. One or two editions prior to the current edition may be kept for loan as indicated by the need and space. No edition of any title shall be kept if its text no longer conforms to current practice. Journals shall be kept according to the Retention Schedule, with no title held longer than twenty years. The entire collection (books, journals, and audiovisuals) shall be reviewed at least annually on a systematic and continuing basis to ensure conformity to the policies given in this document. Materials not conforming to this policy shall be removed from the collection and sold, exchanged, given to other institutions, or destroyed.

Other Resources:

This library has reciprocal agreements with other hospital libraries in Long Beach to make materials available at no cost. Those hospital libraries are at Pacific Hospital, St. Mary Medical Center, Long Beach Veterans Administration Hospital, and the Navy Regional Medical Center. For journal articles not available at those libraries the NLM DOCLINE system is used to make requests and the MLGSCA coupons are used for payment. When articles are not available in a hospital participating in the MLGSCA coupon system, the DOCLINE system automatically routes the request to one of the resource libraries (UCLA, USC, UCI, Loma Linda, UCSD) or to the National Library of Medicine.

Multiple Copies:

No multiple copies of books will be purchased for the Library. Only one subscription will be maintained for each journal in the collection. Additional copies of texts and reference books shall be purchased for nursing stations, offices and laboratories upon request from the head of the department involved and, with approval, charged to the department's budget.

Appendix B

Representative Special Setting Collection Development Policies

The collection development policies which follow are reprinted, with permission of the issuing institutions, from Collection Development Policies for Health Sciences Libraries, compiled by David H. Morse and Daniel T. Richards (Chicago: Medical Library Association, 1992). They illustrate the types of policies which can be developed to guide collection development in settings described in Chapter 7: Selection in Special Settings.

EXAMPLES OF COLLECTION DEVELOPMENT POLICIES FOR A REFER-
ENCE COLLECTION:

THOMAS JEFFERSON UNIVERSITY (PHILADELPHIA, PA)
SCOTT MEMORIAL LIBRARY

Reference Collections

This is a non-circulating collection because of the nature of its materials and use,
with only a few titles duplicated in other collections. Reference tools are distinguished from other materials in the following ways: 1) they are used for consultation
rather than in-depth study; 2) they are often used to provide brief, factual ready
reference information; 3) they are often best used with the assistance of a librarian
since they often require interpretation.

The selection of Reference material is the responsibility of the Information Services
Librarian in charge of the Reference collection in consultation with the Collection
Development Librarian and the Associate Director for Collection Management.

1. Serials Resources
   Scope:
   > a. Standard directories
   > b. Union lists
   > c. Title abbreviations lists

   Retention:
   > Library keeps the latest edition only except when older materials are valuable
   > for verification or location of titles (e.g. *New Serial Titles, World List of Scientific
   > Periodicals*)

2. Book Catalogs
   Scope:
   > a. *Books in Print* series
   > b. MEDOC
   > c. Miscellaneous directories of publishers and specialty publications

   Retention:
   > Only current BIP items are in Reference. Older editions are retired to Acqui-
   > sitions. MEDOC is complete. Miscellaneous publications are retained as long
   > as they are useful.

3. AIDS References
   Scope:
   > Includes works which compile expert opinions, research policies, statistics or
   > projections on various aspects of the epidemic. Any reference tool, such as a
   > handbook or directory, which relates to AIDS is shelved here.

Retention:
The collection will be monitored for currency on an on-going basis. Older material of value will be transferred to the stacks. Superseded publications will be withdrawn.

4. Encyclopedias:
Scope:
Three general knowledge encyclopedias are available as well as authoritative encyclopedias in general science, the social sciences, humanities and biomedical sciences.

Retention:
Only the most current edition owned will be kept in the Library.

5. Dictionaries:
Scope:
a. English language — classics plus several current "college" dictionaries.
b. Subject oriented — most reputable dictionaries in medicine and nursing.
c. Foreign language — English-foreign dictionaries are not acquired. Because these materials are expensive and infrequently used, this collection is limited.
d. Nomenclature and terminology.
e. Quotations lists.

Retention:
Latest editions, classic editions, or currently useful dictionaries are kept in Reference. Most recently superseded editions and little used foreign dictionaries are placed in the stacks. Others are withdrawn.

6. Drug and Toxicology Resources:
Scope:
Drug-oriented and toxicity-oriented materials are both available. American drug handbooks are acquired, with some selection on the basis of currency, uniqueness of content or arrangement, and authoritativeness. Encyclopedic English-language drug resource materials from selected foreign countries are acquired.

Retention:
Official U.S. drug compendia, and other key sources providing substantive content of potential historical usefulness are kept. The latest editions are kept in Reference, with earlier volumes in the stacks. Only the most current edition of other U.S. works and foreign publications are retained; outdated or superseded volumes are withdrawn.

7. Bibliographies:
   Scope:
   Comprehensive, historical bibliographies of current user interest that provide easier or better access to the information included than other available sources are kept in Reference at the discretion of the Reference staff. The availability of online databases limits the necessity to acquire many bibliographies.

   Retention:
   Outdated bibliographies are transferred to the stacks or withdrawn.

8. Meetings and Translations:
   Scope:
   Standard indexes of meetings and/or proceedings in medicine, the sciences and social sciences are acquired.

   Retention:
   Meeting sources are retained for the current two years. Complete runs of proceedings are maintained in Reference as long as their usefulness warrants and space permits.

9. Directories:
   Scope:
   Current directories are acquired which list organizations, societies, institutions, companies, scholarships, educational programs or agencies in:
      a. Biomedical and health fields — local, state, national. International directories are acquired very selectively due to their expense and infrequent use.
      b. Social Sciences — local, state, national directories are selectively acquired.

   Retention:
   Superseded editions are withdrawn.

10. Biographical Directories:
    Scope:
    Current directories are collected in many fields:
       a. Notables: national and international.
       b. Scientists: national and international.
       c. Biomedical and health sciences: all major directories collected.
    Membership lists of individual medical societies and associations are acquired selectively since the information in them is often less complete than that in standard directories. Such lists are acquired in related fields to help fill gaps in standard directories.

    Retention:
    Only the current editions of general directories, except for major historical cumulated sources, are kept. Standard directories of medical specialists are

kept permanently. The most recent edition is kept in Reference with earlier editions shelved in the stacks. Membership lists of specialty societies or organizations are retained only when they contain useful biographical information.

11. Handbooks and Style Manuals:
    Scope:
    Titles in all core subjects (biomedical sciences and clinical specialties) and selected titles in physical and social sciences are collected. General reference works such as almanacs, etiquette books and some government handbooks are included. Also found here are guides to the literature, style manuals and writing guides.
    Retention:
    Only the most current edition of each title is kept in Reference. The most recently superseded editions are transferred to the stacks. Clinical handbooks are withdrawn when a copy already is in the stacks. Superseded almanacs are withdrawn.

12. Statistical Resources
    Scope:
    Publications, including serials from U.S. government agencies or official bodies containing significant statistical compilations of data on health care, morbidity and mortality, socioeconomic factors related to health or disease are acquired. Major studies which are comprised primarily of relevant statistical data will be placed in the Reference collection. Studies which include substantial narrative discussion should be placed in the circulating collection. Major sources of international health, health manpower or disease-related data are acquired.

    Retention:
    Most series are kept indefinitely in Reference as space permits. Less significant publications and those dealing with specific subjects not of current importance are transferred to the stacks when their usefulness declines.

13. Standards and Codes
    Scope:
    Practice standards, codes of ethics and standards for accreditation of programs/facilities relevant to the health sciences professions. Legal materials on this topic are kept in Section 16 (Legal Resources).

    Retention:
    Usually only current editions remain in Reference. Older editions of some AMA publication are retained in Reference for convenience.

14. History of Medicine
    Scope:
    A small collection of tools for ready reference in the history of medicine and
    nursing including origin of terms and eponyms.

    Retention:
    Materials are of non-current nature and are kept in Reference indefinitely.

15. Test and Measurements
    Scope:
    Standard reference bibliographies and indexes to tests and measurements are
    shelved here. No attempt is made to collect actual copies of tests.

    Retention:
    All volumes of ongoing series are maintained in Reference. For works where
    new editions do not entirely supersede previous editions, several older edi-
    tions are maintained in Reference. Completely outdated material is with-
    drawn from the collection rather than being transferred to the stacks.

16. Legal Resources
    Scope:
    a.Official compendia of legislative or administrative law restricted to health-
    related sections when possible, are acquired for U.S. and Pennsylvania.
    b.Regulations and standards issued by major health-related organizations are
    acquired when available.

    Retention:
    In general only those laws and standards currently in effect are kept.

17. Grants Resources
    Scope:
    Foundation directories—local, national and international; and a wide variety
    of lists of grants and awards given, mainly federal. Nine serials relating to
    grants are shelved here:
      Aris Funding Messenger
      Federal Grants and Contracts Weekly
      Foundation Grants Alert
      Foundation Grants Index Quarterly
      Foundation News
      Grants Magazine
      Health Funds Development Letter
      Medical Research Funding Bulletin
      NIH Guide for Grants and Contracts

    Retention:
    The latest edition only of this material is kept with older material being
    withdrawn. Material judged to be of continuing interest, such as the PHS and

NIH Grants series, are kept indefinitely. Serial publications are kept from one to three years according to title.

18. Geographical and Travel Resources
   Scope:
      a. Atlases—state, national, international.
      b. Gazetteers.
      c. Travel guides (e.g. *OAG Travel Planner, Hotel and Motel Red Book*)

   Retention:
   Only current editions are kept.

JOHNS HOPKINS UNIVERSITY (BALTIMORE, MD)
WILLIAM H. WELCH MEDICAL LIBRARY

REFERENCE COLLECTION

STATEMENT OF PURPOSE:
The Welch Reference Collection is a core collection of highly-used general and specialized sources of information. Items in the reference collection are selected because they support the teaching, research, patient care, and administrative activities of the faculty, students, and staff at the Johns Hopkins Medical Institutions. Titles are included in this collection primarily because they provide access to the journal literature (indexes, abstracts, and compact disk databases); provide factual information (directories, handbooks, dictionaries, and statistical compilations); or give general background information on a topic (encyclopedias and textbooks). The collection is arranged in 15 subject sections; a description of each section follows. Since the purpose of the Reference Collection is to serve immediate and specific needs, the material is non-circulating and with the exception of medical textbooks, is generally not duplicated elsewhere in the collection. Two smaller reference collections exist. The Psychiatry/Neurosciences Library has a reference collection whose focus is on psychiatry, neurology, and the neurosciences, and the Oncology Center Library has a small reference collection which includes the most important sources in the field of oncology.

INDEXES AND ABSTRACTS:
Overview:
Indexes and abstracts are collected in the clinical and basic sciences, and in peripheral areas which are of general interest (for example, indexes to medical and scientific meetings). Whenever possible, alternative formats for the indexes and abstracts will be identified and evaluated.

Retention Statement:
As a general rule, all volumes of the indexes and abstracts should be retained. Exceptions may arise due to low use, shortage of stack space, or because the index or abstract is available in an electronic format. The exceptions should be addressed on a case-by-case basis.

SUBJECT SECTIONS: (Note: Authoritative sources marked by an * are listed at the end of this document.)
    Section 1: Encyclopedias and Geographical Sources
        Overview:
            One general encyclopedia will be available as well as any authoritative encyclopedias in scientific or biomedical areas. The encyclopedias should not be more than five years old, unless the title has been identified as a standard encyclopedia in the field according to an authoritative source*, or it contains information that will not change with time. This section will include a few current, basic, and concise geographic sources and almanacs containing vital information about the United States and the rest of the world. Finally, current phone directories for London, Paris, and Rome will be available. Phone directories for other U.S. cities are collected on microfiche only.

        Retention Statement:
            Include current editions of encyclopedias only in Section 1. Earlier editions of general encyclopedias should be discarded.

            Retain the most recent edition of the almanacs and geographical sources in this section; older editions should be discarded. Retain the current year only of the phone books; discard when replaced with a new edition.

    Section 2: Dictionaries/Abbreviations/Nomenclature/Classification
        Overview:
            Dictionaries related to science, biomedicine, social sciences, and selected areas of the chemical and physical sciences will be selected for this section. There will also be a substantial collection of foreign language dictionaries which can include general, scientific, or medical information.

        Retention Statement:
            Retain most recent editions only in Section 2; older editions of medical and health-related materials may be moved to the general collection. Older editions of dictionaries whose subjects are peripheral will be discarded. Only the most current works in abbreviations, nomenclature, and classification should be retained; older editions will be moved to the general collection.

    Section 3: Writing Guides
        Overview:
            General style manuals, authoritative works on writing for publication and manuals used by special organizations or publications related to healthcare or behavioral sciences will be available. This section also includes several works on writing resumes, cover letters, and curriculum vitae.

Retention Statement:
Retain current editions only. Older editions of specialized material may be discarded. Authoritative writing manuals or guides may be kept indefinitely in the general collection.

Section 4: People/Societies/Organizations
Overview:
Biographical directories for international and U.S. notables, especially those with an emphasis in science and biomedicine will be available. Current membership directories for health-care organizations, medical and scientific societies will also be included in this section.

Retention Statement:
Retain current edition of organizational membership directories, societies, institutions, or corporations, international and U.S., which are related to the biomedical or health-care fields. Older copies will be housed in the general collection. Older editions of general directories will be discarded. Membership directories will not be retained at all unless they contain biographical information.

Section 5: Library and Information Sources
Overview:
Directories of librarians, libraries, information centers and organizational memberships, and information pertinent to the publishing industry are appropriate sources for this section. Specialized subject guides to the literature in the basic and clinical sciences will be available whenever possible.

Retention Statement:
Retain current editions of directories, subject guides to the literature, handbooks, reference sources, and publishing information. Older editions with historical value will reside in the general collection. Older editions of most subject guides to the literature will be discarded.

Section 6: Handbooks
Overview:
Standard, authoritative handbooks in the basic and clinical sciences should be selected for this section. The handbooks should contain statistical tables, graphs, standard equations and other important mathematical equations.

Retention Statement:
Retain current handbooks in core subjects related to basic sciences, clinical sciences, and selected works in the physical or social sciences. Earlier editions will be housed in the general collection. Works in peripheral areas may be discarded.

Section 7: Statistical Sources
Overview:
This section should include current U.S. government and other official publications containing statistical information on health care, vital statistics, and socio-economic issues related to health care. Similar materials for the state of Maryland which are data- or fact-oriented will also be selected for this section. A few general statistical compilations should also be available.

Retention Statement:
Previous editions of statistical publications may be housed in the general collection. Older editions of general statistical compilations should be discarded.

Section 8: Funding Sources
Overview:
Current sources of grants, awards, loans and scholarships from various sources including private foundations and the U.S. government are appropriate for this section. Both general and biomedical sources should be available.

Retention Statement:
Previous editions should be discarded. Sources which are older than three years (and no current edition is available) should be removed from this section and discarded.

Section 9: Educational Information
Overview:
This section should include sources of current information about medical schools worldwide, graduate medical education and training programs, medical licensure, and statistics on matching programs. A few significant sources of information about undergraduate schools should also be available. Medical school catalogs are available on microfiche.

Retention Statement:
Older editions are discarded. Current catalogs of other U.S. medical schools are maintained on fiche only.

Section 10: Medical Textbooks
Overview:
This section should include the most current, significant textbooks in the basic and clinical sciences. Selection of these titles is based on faculty or staff recommendations, recommended lists for medical libraries*, and book reviews published in medical journals. Items selected for this section should closely match the student reserve collection housed in the Pre-Clinical Teaching Building.

Retention Statement:
One copy of the current edition and all previous editions will be placed in the general collection.

Section 11: Pharmacology and Toxicology
Overview:
Authoritative drug information sources required for patient care and research will be selected for this section. Compendia and pharmacopoeias from foreign countries are acquired whenever available. Current sources of toxicology information also reside here. Product catalogs from pharmaceutical companies are not kept in reference.

Retention Statement:
Older editions will be housed in the general collection.

Section 12: Scientific Supplies/Research Facilities/Hospitals & Clinics
Overview:
A core collection of current catalogs and directories associated with medical or health-related manufacturers, equipment, and supplies should be available. This section will also include national and international directories of hospitals, research facilities, clinics and other health care centers.

Retention Statement:
This section should include current directories only. Previous editions should be discarded. Sources older than three years are out of date and should be removed from this section and discarded.

Section 13: Legal and Government Information Sources
Overview:
This section should include laws governing the practice of medicine in Maryland as well as any national regulations that apply to Maryland physicians, including the health-related portion of the Maryland Annotated Code.

Retention Statement:
Retain all official and regulatory information relating to health care. Everything in this section is current; older items will be discarded.

Section 14: Computers
Overview:
This section should include a core collection of current, standard, comprehensive reference directories of computer software and hardware. Emphasis is on sources related to health care, database searching, information technology, and microcomputer hardware systems that the Library supports.

Retention Statement:
Previous editions should be discarded. Sources older than three years are out-of-date and should be removed from this section and discarded.

Section 15: Hopkins and Baltimore Information
Overview:
This section will include significant works detailing the history associated with the Johns Hopkins Medical Institutions as well as books about Baltimore which include some mention of the medical complex. The section may contain one or two texts on the history of medicine; however, in-depth historical information is available in the Institute of the History of Medicine.

Retention Statement:
Retain all significant works, regardless of date of publication.

EXAMPLE OF A COLLECTION DEVELOPMENT POLICY FOR AN
AUDIOVISUAL COLLECTION:

COLUMBIA UNIVERSITY (NEW YORK, NY)
AUGUSTUS C. LONG HEALTH SCIENCES LIBRARY

AUDIOVISUALS

I. BACKGROUND:
In June 1973, the Columbia University College of Physicians and Surgeons was
awarded a grant from the National Library of Medicine for the establishment of
a "prototypical multimedia facility." This grant represented the initial attention
paid to the integration of audiovisual and other non-print materials into the
Health Sciences Library collections. The award was used to demonstrate the uses
of media in a library setting, establishing precedent for a much larger media area
in the planning and construction of a new library facility.

The Health Sciences Library moved to its current site in the Hammer Health
Sciences Center in 1976. The Media Center occupies approximately 12,000 sq. ft.
on the second floor of the Library, and the perimeter of the Media Center has
remained constant. The original design emphasized generous areas for shelving
and viewing media materials, catering to individual, small, and large class-size
group use. A service area with room for library staff activities and a media reserve
collection were also both part of the original design that has remained until the
present.

Significant change has occurred, however, in the physical layout and arrangement within the Media Center facility. In 1986, approximately 20% of the Media
Center was remodeled to create a microcomputer laboratory which provided a
setting for computer-based instruction and public access microcomputing for the
users of the Health Sciences Library. In 1988, an additional 20% of the Media
Center was remodeled and equipped as a microcomputer classroom for computer-based instruction. This was made possible by supplemental funding from
the four Health Sciences Schools and by an equipment grant from a computer
manufacturer. In 1990, the Medical School's Alumni Association obtained a
cardiology patient simulator, which is housed in an area formerly used for
small-group viewing of media materials. These changes not only account for the
busy public services atmosphere of the Media Center, but also have demonstrated the need for a dynamic and progressive collection development policy.

II. DESCRIPTION OF THE COLLECTION:
**Note: General interest computer software and programming languages are
considered part of microcomputer collection development.**

The collections of the Health Sciences Library Media Center are unique within
the Columbia University Libraries and are considered a regional resource within
the cooperative networks in which the Health Sciences Library participates.

The collection consists of approximately 6,000 items in the following formats: 35mm slide, audiocassette, 3/4" (u-matic) and 1/2" (VHS) videocassette, 35mm filmstrip, microforms (film and fiche), interactive laser videodiscs, models, simulators, realia, and computer-assisted instruction programs, and authoring tools (IBM, Macintosh, and Apple II formats).

In addition to the non-print materials in the Media Center's collection, print materials are acquired to support use and research related to non-print materials. Selected periodicals which focus on audiovisual or computer topics are also maintained on a reference basis.

A wide variety of materials geared to health science students and professionals is represented in the Media Center's collections. Areas of strength include materials directly supporting the curriculum of biomedical programs, such as human gross anatomy, neuroanatomy, physical assessment, human growth and development, orthopedics, and psychiatry. Many clinical specialties in medicine, nursing, dentistry, and physical therapy are also represented by the Media Center's holdings. These include physical examination and diagnosis, psychotherapy, internal medicine, obstetrics, neonatal care, and sexually transmitted diseases. Videotape and slide materials focusing on both the health-care and pathologic implications of acquired immune deficiency syndrome (AIDS) are also well represented in the Media Center's holdings.

In support of continuing education efforts, the Media Center subscribes to audiovisual serials, such as the Network for Continuing Medical Education's videocassette programs and the Audio Digest Foundation's audiocassettes on clinical specialties.

The Media Center, generally, does not collect patient education and health information materials, given the non-lay orientation of our primary clientele. However, materials which consistently support curricular and clinical programs are collected. Except for materials related to occupational and physical therapies, programs created for allied health professionals or students are not collected.

III. COOPERATIVE ARRANGEMENTS:
The Media Center participates in a collection development grant program administered by the Hospital Library Services Program of the New York Metropolitan Reference and Research Library Agency (METRO). This annual grant funds the purchase of audiovisual materials that become part of the Library's normal collection, with the stipulation that the materials will physically return to METRO if and when an institution closes or is unable to support cooperative access to the materials through interlibrary loan.

All non-reserve media materials are borrowable by other institutions according to normal interlibrary loan procedures administered through the Regional Medical Library system.

IV. CRITERIA AND GUIDELINES FOR COLLECTION DEVELOPMENT:

The primary function of the Media Center is to support the education mission of Columbia University's Health Sciences Division. In contrast with the research-oriented mission of the Health Sciences Library as a whole, the Media Center's collection development policy reflects a unique biomedical instructional orientation. Therefore, criteria applied to audiovisual materials differ from the overall criteria applied to other Library collections.

Rather than an adopting an archival or research orientation, the primary emphasis is placed on the relevance to the actual or anticipated needs of the users in the Health Sciences educational and clinical programs. Selection depends upon initiating and cultivating working relationships with the faculty and staff of the various schools and educational units. Awareness and knowledge of trends and developments in biomedical education and instructional technology are also important prerequisites for establishing a useful and relevant collection.

Audiovisual collection development is both reactive and proactive. Input from users is an important means of discovering collection weaknesses and new developments in the curriculum. The selector must take an active role in discovering and evaluating new materials and technologies and promoting their value. This should include exploration of techniques and resources which have not been previously tried, subject to an evaluation period to decide on permanent, ongoing support.

The criteria employed by the selector of health sciences audiovisual materials ideally should conform to the guidelines developed by a working group comprised of representatives from the Association of American Medical Colleges, the Association of Biomedical Communications Directors, the National Audiovisual Center, and others. [See Attributes of Quality in Audiovisual Materials for Health Professionals. Journal of Biocommunications. July 1981; 8(2): 5-11]. The basic categories of evaluation in this set of guidelines include content, instructional design, technical production, and packaging. Within each broad category are specific suggestions of points of evaluation or comparison which transcend differences in particular formats or media. Combined with an in-depth understanding of the Media Center's needs and the needs of users, the selector has a significant tool for building a relevant and useful collection.

Previews and experimental trials of new media materials should be pursued whenever possible. Limitations to a mandatory preview policy include the inability of suppliers to provide preview copies, expense, and the limited time constraints of faculty to participate in a meaningful preview or trial.

V. DESELECTION:

Deselection is particularly important for maintaining the collection's relevance to the educational and clinical programs within the Medical Center. Deselection (weeding) of audiovisual materials is done on an item-by-item basis. Important considerations are outdated or inaccurate content, conspicuous deviation from current health practice or therapy, deteriorated format, and format obsolescence.

**EXAMPLE OF A COLLECTION DEVELOPMENT POLICY FOR A CON-
SUMER HEALTH COLLECTION:**

*DARTMOUTH COLLEGE (HANOVER, NH)
BIOMEDICAL LIBRARIES*

CONSUMER HEALTH COLLECTION
Purpose of the collection:
   The Consumer Health Collection exists to serve users seeking authoritative
   information, in clearly understood language, about diseases, conditions, treatments, and other health care topics of interest to consumers of health care.

User groups:
   Dartmouth Medical School students - materials to help explain health and
   disease concepts to patients and families; materials in support of Partners in
   Health Education program.

   Dartmouth Medical School faculty - materials to help explain health and disease
   concepts to patients and families.

   Dartmouth-Hitchcock Medical Center personnel - materials to help explain
   health and disease concepts to patients and families, materials for personal use.

   Dartmouth-Hitchcock Medical Center patients, families, and visitors - materials
   on health and disease. (These users may not check material out.)

   Dartmouth College personnel - materials on health and disease.

   Members of the community at large - materials on health and disease. (These
   users may not check material out.)

Scope of the collection:
   The Consumer Health Collection will provide selected and authoritative written
   and audiovisual material intended to inform health care consumers about specific diseases and conditions, treatment options, medications, and problems of
   coping with chronic diseases. Materials on basic wellness and nutrition will also
   be collected, but those advocating specific weight-reduction diets and exercise
   programs will generally not be included. A representative selection of material
   on alternative medicine may be collected for informational purposes, but those
   advocating specific alternative therapeutics will generally not be included.

Subjects:
   In the following subject areas, a small number of current, authoritative, and
   comprehensive titles will be collected, e.g. *The Family Mental Health Encyclopedia*.
   In addition, one or more titles will be collected on specific common diseases
   and/or treatments, e.g. *How to Cope With Depression*:

Allergy & Clinical Immunology	Neurology
Cardiology	Obstetrics & Gynecology
Connective Tissue Disease	Ophthalmology
Dermatology	Otolaryngology
Endocrinology & Metabolism	Pediatrics & Adolescent
Gastroenterology	Medicine
General Internal Medicine	Physical Medicine &
Genetics & Perinatal Medicine	Rehabilitation
Geriatrics	Psychiatry
Hematology & Oncology	Pulmonary Disease
Infectious Disease	Radiation Oncology
Nephrology & Hypertension	Surgery

In the following subject areas, only a few current, authoritative, and comprehensive titles will be collected. Works on specific diseases, conditions, and treatments will generally not be included:

Alternative Medicine	Nutrition
Anatomy	Pathology
Anesthesiology	Radiology
Clinical Pharmacology	Wellness
Health Care System	

Criteria for selection:
The following criteria are used to select material for the Consumer Health Collection:

1. Need - lack of similar titles, demand
2. Appropriateness - subject fits into the scope of the collection
3. Qualifications of the Author - relevant academic credentials, publications record, authoritative institutional affiliations
4. Content - significance, accuracy, balance, documentation, authority, timeliness
5. Presentation - quality of writing, style, readability
6. Ease of Use - organization, presence of indexes, table of contents
7. Pathways to Further Information - bibliographies, reading lists, referral sources, resource organizations
8. Physical Quality - size of type, clarity of print, aesthetic appeal, binding, durability
9. Consumer Orientation - appropriateness for lay use, usefulness for making informed decisions concerning health and medical services
10. Language - English language only

(Adapted from: Alan M. Rees and Catherine Hoffman, *Consumer Health Information Source Book*, 3rd ed., Oryx Press, 1990.)

Formats:
> Books will be the primary format collected. Videotapes, journals, and other formats may also be collected.

Reference materials:
> A few dictionaries, encyclopedias, and directories are included in the Consumer Health Collection. More extensive reference resources are available in the Matthews-Fuller Health Sciences Library's professional reference collection.

> Indexes to consumer health literature will be available in print and computerized formats. *Health Reference Center*, a CD-ROM-based consumer health information resource, provides access to an extensive collection of journal articles and pamphlets through both indexing and full-text.

Currency of the collection:
> Currency of the collection will be maintained through a regular program of selection, acquisition, and weeding. Because the focus of the collection is current, authoritative material, most materials will have been published within the last five years. Items older than five years will be reviewed periodically to determine their continued usefulness in the collection.

Responsibility for selection:
> The Health Sciences Librarian will have responsibility for selection of materials for the Consumer Health Collection. Selection will be based on reviews in the professional library literature, such as *Library Journal*, and/or recommendations from Dartmouth-Hitchcock Medical Center consumer/patient health education providers.

Relationships to other collections:
> Other local resources of consumer health information include the Parenting Library and the Cancer Library, both at the Dartmouth-Hitchcock Medical Center; the Women's Health Resource Center; and the Howe Library, Lebanon Public Library, and other public libraries.

6/94

EXAMPLES OF COLLECTION DEVELOPMENT POLICIES FOR A HISTORI-
CAL COLLECTION:

COLUMBIA UNIVERSITY (NEW YORK, NY)
AUGUSTUS C. LONG HEALTH SCIENCES LIBRARY

RARE BOOKS AND SPECIAL COLLECTIONS

I. INTRODUCTION:
The Library's collections in the histories of health sciences are significant ones,
and, in many cases, are considered of national as well as regional importance.
Though a systematic analysis of the entire collection has not been completed,
comparisons of holdings in selected areas with the 4th edition (1983) of *A Medical
Bibliography: An Annotated Checklist of Texts Illustrating the History of Medicine*
(Garrison and Morton), the standard bibliography of "firsts" in all areas of the
health sciences, have demonstrated that the Health Sciences Library frequently
holds more than 75% of the items listed. The Library's rare books and special
collections are managed by the Special Collections Librarian.

The Special Collections Section contains more than 12,000 rare and historical
books, a like number of periodical volumes, and large collections of pamphlets,
pictures and portraits, artifacts, and archival records in all areas of the health
sciences. A large portion of the collection has been added through routine
acquisition, but three private libraries, those of George Sumner Huntington, M.D.
(1861-1927), John Green Curtis, M.D. (1844-1913), and Jerome Pierce Webster,
M.D. (1888-1974), form its core. Other collections of note are the Lena and Louis
Hyman Collection in the History of Anesthesia, the June Lyday and Samuel T.
Orton Collection on dyslexia, the Auchincloss Collection of Florence Nightingale
letters and memorabilia, the William J. Gies Archive on Dental Education, and
an extensive collection of Columbia-Presbyterian Medical Center publications
and memorabilia. The Library's rare book collection includes nearly every
edition of the works of Vesalius, Harvey, and Tagliacozzi; twenty-three incunabula; and many of the classics in the history of medicine.

The historical collection as a whole is among the 10 best national collections in
the health sciences, comparing favorably with the historical collections of Johns
Hopkins and UCLA, but lacking the comprehensiveness of those at Yale,
Countway (Harvard), the New York Academy of Medicine, and the National
Library of Medicine. The strengths of this collection are many but are less well
known than those of some of our counterparts. Especially important items in the
collection include:

- One of only 13 recorded copies (completely restored in 1981) of the
  1543 Epitome of Vesalius' great anatomy. HSL is the only library in the
  world holding 4 copies of the first edition of the Fabrica;

- Thomas Geminus' plagiarized edition of the Fabrica, which Geminus
  issued as his own in London, 1553, containing the famous Adam &
  Eve nudes;

- A manuscript record book from the Pharmacy of St. Paul in Bologna, which contains prescriptions signed by Tagliacozzi and Aldrovandi. The signature of Tagliacozzi is the only recorded one in the U.S.;

- The autographed presentation copy to Charles Lennox, the Duke of Richmond, of Joseph Carpue's 1816 *An Account of Two Successful Operations for Restoring a Lost Nose*, the work which marks the emergence of modern plastic surgery;

- One of only eight sets of the life size anatomical engravings of Ercole Lelli, done in 1780, mounted on linen;

- Florence Nightingale's Bible and several hundred of her letters.

The uncataloged backlog includes approximately 3,000 rare books from the 16th century forward, several hundred prints and photographs, and manuscript material relating to the history of the Medical Center. Additionally, there are a few smaller archival collections, including the personal archive of Viola W. Bernard, M.D.; the publishing archive relating to Charles May's classic textbook on ophthalmology; and a collection of student lecture notes from the early days of the Medical faculty of Columbia University and the College of Physicians & Surgeons.

A large support collection of works relating to the history of the health sciences is maintained as a part of the Library's open stack collection. These materials include bibliographies, biographies, book catalogs of medical historical collections throughout the world, directories, dictionaries, and encyclopedias; as well as books about books, bibliography, and printing history. The collection development policy for secondary material in the history of the health sciences is detailed in the general collection development policy for the library.

II. NAMED COLLECTIONS:

The following named collections demonstrate the depth, scope, and subject focus of the overall collections:

The **Jerome P. Webster Library of Plastic Surgery** was maintained as a separate library until the opening of the new Health Sciences Library in 1976. Jerome P. Webster was a renowned plastic surgeon, historian, and faculty member at P&S from 1928 until his death in 1974. He assembled an extensive library of both historical and contemporary works in plastic surgery. The Library's collection also includes patient records, graphics, and correspondence. (A printed brochure describing this collection is available.)

The **Huntington Collection** contains approximately 1,000 books in early anatomy and comparative anatomy, assembled by George Sumner Huntington, Chairman of the Department of Anatomy at the College of Physicians & Surgeons from 1889 to 1925. After his death, the collection was purchased with funds raised by the Huntington Memorial Committee, a group of P&S alumni and faculty.

This work was restored in 1981. An especially fine feature of the collection is the large number of anatomical atlases.

The **Curtis Collection,** similar in size to the Huntington Collection, was assembled by John Green Curtis, Chairman of the Department of Physiology at P&S. It contains early editions of Aristotle, Hippocrates, Galen, and Harvey, and other works important in the history of physiology, with the histories of histology and embryology particularly well represented.

The **Memorabilia Collection** is a growing collection of publications and manuscript materials about or emanating from the institutions, faculties, or individuals associated with the Columbia-Presbyterian Medical Center. The Collection includes, but is not limed to, bulletins, yearbooks, reports of the Deans, minutes of faculty and committee meetings, course syllabi, student lecture notes, early grade reports, patient records, theses and dissertations, occasional artifacts, bound collected reprints from some divisions and departments, and works published about the institution or by individuals with some institutional association. Though the collection has considerable archival holdings and runs of official publications, it has never achieved the status of an institutional archive, nor is that the Library's purpose.

The **Lena and Louis Hyman Collection in the History of Anesthesia** is the Library's newest collection, having been established in 1982. This collection of one hundred thirty-three works related to the development of modern anesthesiology was presented to the Health Sciences Library by Allen I. Hyman, M.D., Professor of Anesthesiology in the College of Physicians & Surgeons.

In 1986, the William J. Gies Foundation established in the Health Sciences Library the **Gies Foundation Archive for the History of Dental Education.** This collection brings together manuscript and published material relating to the history of dental education in the United States, especially as it was developed at Columbia by Gies, William B. and Dunning, Henry S.

The Library's collection in the history of dentistry contains many of the important works in the history of dentistry. Early dental journals record the advance of dentistry and form, in many ways, the primary literature for the science. The Library's collection of dental journals is extensive and contains especially strong holdings of nineteenth-century American titles. The Library also has a significant collection of nineteenth-century monographs, including those in the Lena and Louis Hyman Collection in the History of Anesthesia. Manuscript materials relating to the history of dentistry in the twentieth-century are included in the M-Collection.

The Special Collections Section has an active interest in the history of nursing. It currently houses **The Auchincloss Collection of Florence Nightingale Letters,** which is a collection of books by and about Florence Nightingale (1820-1910), various items of Nightingale memorabilia, and nearly 300 letters in Miss Nightingale's hand. The nucleus of this collection was a gift from Hugh Auchincloss, M.D., attending surgeon at the Presbyterian Hospital and Professor of Clinical Surgery, College of Physicians & Surgeons. It has since been enhanced by gifts from the Nursing alumnae.

The Library also has an active program to acquire classic nursing textbooks of the 19th and early 20th centuries, as well as a broad representation of source works on the history of American nursing practice.

The **Sigmund Freud Library** contains approximately half of the book collection which Freud left behind when he fled Vienna with his family in 1938. Many volumes have been annotated by Freud. The provenance of the collection was confirmed by Anna Freud during a visit to the Library in 1976.

The **June Lyday and Samuel T. Orton Collection** contains approximately 4,000 case records of the Orton's patients, patients with dyslexia and other learning disorders. Dr. Samuel T. Orton was a graduate of P&S, was the founder of the Orton Society, and was the first to diagnose dyslexia. (A printed brochure describing this collection is available.)

III. OTHER AREAS:
Although the scope of the collection is comprehensive, the Library's collection development program has in recent years given emphasis to the following subjects and disciplines:

- The history of biochemistry;
- The development of immunochemistry in the twentieth-century;
- Social aspects of medicine;
- The history of neurology;
- The history of oncology; and
- The history of pediatrics.

IV. COOPERATIVE ARRANGEMENTS:
An attempt is made to initiate purchases which do not duplicate holdings in other institutions in the metropolitan area. Similarly, gifts are frequently referred to other institutions whose special interests are known. The Health Sciences Library has an informal cooperative arrangement with The New York Academy of Medicine Library, the only other history of the health sciences collection of particular note in New York City. Cooperative programs for preservation of historical collections are under discussion within the Research Libraries Group and the National Library of Medicine.

V. CRITERIA AND GUIDELINES FOR COLLECTION DEVELOPMENT:
There is no systematic academic or research program in the history of the health sciences, nor is there likelihood of one in the future. The primary clientele of Special Collections is distributed throughout the Columbia University commu-

nity, and extends to other institutions throughout the world. Consequently, the collection development policy builds on established strengths rather than anticipated future needs.

The major strengths in the book collections are noted above. As material is available on the market, and is within the limits of our budget, items may be acquired.

The selection criteria (i.e., relevance to actual needs of Columbia's educational, research, or clinical programs; scope and content; depth of the existing collection; quality; price; language and country of origin) which are applied to materials for the regular collection are also applied generally in decisions for rare and historical materials. Additional factors which may be considered or which may assume a greater importance in making a selection decision include the following:

- the presence of other editions of the same work;
- the availability of a facsimile edition;
- the association value of the item;
- price;
- physical condition;
- artifactual characteristics, e.g. fine binding, autographs;
- provenance; and
- local availability.

The selection decision is usually made by applying all relevant criteria, and rarely will a single factor determine the decision. Gifts of rare or unique materials in most health science areas are accepted under the same selecting guidelines.

The Library has a small but growing program for acquisition of archival and manuscript materials. A substantial collection already exists in the Memorabilia Collection, and some smaller individual collections have been accepted, with accompanying funds to cover processing costs. As of 1985, an effort has been made to acquire two copies of all publications of all Medical Center institutions, one copy being an archival copy deposited in Special Collections. The other copy is added to the stack collection. Biographies about people who have had important associations with CPMC, and other materials about the Medial Center, are actively solicited and collected.

The transfer of all pre-1876 material from the open stacks to the Special Collections stacks is currently underway. Other items are routinely identified for transfer to this collection as well; these may include serials or monographs which are important historically.

COLLEGE OF PHYSICIANS (PHILADELPHIA, PA)
LIBRARY

B. Historical Services Division (pre-1966):

Established in 1953 to make the Library's rare book, manuscript, archival, and print and photograph collections accessible to scholars and to provide a specialized focus for their acquisition, utilization, and preservation, the Library's Historical Services Division houses one of the finest history of medicine collections in the world. The Historical Services Division of the Library contains over 220,000 monographs and bound serials published before 1966. More than 400 are incunabula, and 12,000 are pre-1801 imprints. There are strong holdings in anatomy, dermatology, embryology, neurology/neurosurgery, obstetrics/gynecology, ophthalmology, and pediatrics, and particularly rich collections in homeopathy, popular medicine, tuberculosis, and yellow fever. The department also consists of the largest collection of William Harvey's works in this country as well as the Joseph T. Freeman Collection of Gerontology and the Samuel D. Gross Library of Surgery.

The manuscript collection (numbering about one million items) is composed of medieval illuminated manuscripts, hundreds of 18th and 19th-century student lecture notes, and the papers of a number of prominent leaders of American medicine, such as Robley Dunglison, S. Weir Mitchell, George B. Wood, Joseph Leidy, W.W. Keen, Charles Harrison Frazier, and Francis C. Wood. The records and archives of medical societies, organizations, and institutions, both extinct and extant, local and national, constitute a major resource for the scholar. The archives of the College of Physicians are important, for the institution has addressed a variety of professional and community concerns since its founding in 1787.

    1. Rare Book Collections (Pre-1900):
      a. Categories:
        Additions to the rare book collection are determined primarily on the basis of strength within the Historical Collections of the Library. The areas in which rare books are collected comprehensively are:

Anatomy	Obstetrics/Gynecology
Cardiology	Ophthalmology
Dermatology	Pediatrics
Embryology	Phrenology
Gerontology	Popular Health
Homeopathy	Public Health
Neurology/	Yellow Fever
Neurosurgery	

        In addition to these areas, additions to the Rare Book Collection are made in the following areas:

1) Sixteenth-century publications in all European languages. Incunabula (pre-1501 imprints) will not be purchased but will be added to the collection if donated.

2) Publications from the seventeenth through the nineteenth-centuries (including journals) are acquired. Emphasis is placed upon British, French, and German imprints relating to those areas of subject strength (see above). Publications from Italy, Spain, and the Scandinavian countries are acquired on a very selective basis.

3) Pre-1850 American imprints (including journals) are collected comprehensively. American imprints from 1850-1900 are collected comprehensively in only those areas identified as collection strengths (see above).

4) Publications relating to Pennsylvania, especially Philadelphia, are collected comprehensively.

5) Pre-1900 Mexican, Central, and South American imprints are collected on a selective basis.

6) Works by William Harvey and Galen are collected comprehensively.

7) American broadsides, advertisements, trade catalogues, medical school announcements and matriculation lists, and annual reports of asylums and hospitals are collected.

b. Selection Guidelines by Format or Type of Material:

1) Academic Dissertations
Academic dissertations are selectively acquired.

2) Bibliographies
Bibliographies pertaining to the history of medicine and allied sciences are actively acquired.

3) Biographies and Autobiographies
Biographies and autobiographies are actively acquired.

4) Catalogs
Catalogs of exhibits relating to the history of medicine and containing items of historical interest are collected.

5) Ephemera

Ephemeral items such as newspaper clippings, announcements, fact sheets, brochures, and posters of historical interest are collected.

6) Festschriften

Festschriften commemorating special events relating to prominent health professionals or institutions are selectively acquired.

7) Foreign Language Materials

Foreign language materials within the scope of the Historical Services Division are collected.

8) Imprint Variants

Materials that are published in two or more places are collected in a single edition with the U.S. edition preferred. However, if the title, preface, or textual contents of the works differ, both imprints are collected. Works printed before 1801 and Americana are exceptions to this rule and may be collected in multiple imprints.

9) Lectures and Speeches

Separately published lectures, speeches, and addresses in core subjects are collected as well as annual orations to medical societies and introductory lectures in medical schools - particularly in the U.S. and Philadelphia.

10) Manuscripts

Manuscripts and transcript collections relating to American medicine from the seventeenth-century to present, with particular emphasis on Pennsylvania and Philadelphia, are actively acquired. European manuscripts are collected only in those areas relating to collection strength.

11) Monographs

Monographs are actively sought in subject areas of collection strength; rare books are collected comprehensively in subject areas listed under Rare Book Collections (Section IV.B.1.a.).

12) Pamphlets

Pamphlets within the scope of the collection are acquired.

13) Portraits (Special)

Original portraits and photographic portraits of physicians, health personnel, and other individuals important to the history of medicine are collected.

14) Prints and Photographs (Special)
Prints and photographs within the scope of the collection are acquired.

15) Reprints
Reprint editions of monographs, series, and serials are collected if the Library lacks the original, if the original held is in poor condition or if it is too valuable to circulate, or if the reprint contains significant material which is lacking in the original edition. Reprints of the collected works of a physician or medical writer which are published in a volume or series are collected. A monographic collection of reprints or a reprint series is generally collected if it relates to a core subject of special importance. Reprints of single journal articles from journals that the Library owns are collected only from 19th-century journals.

16) Textbooks
Pre-1900 textbooks are collected with emphasis on relevant subject areas.

17) Translations
Translations from a foreign language into English are collected when appropriate. Translations from English into a foreign language are not collected except when the work is of exceptional historical interest, contains significant added material, or was printed before 1900.

2. Book/Pamphlet Collection (1900-1965):
   a. Categories:
   Acquisitions in this area are actively sought only in those areas of collection strength (see Rare Book Collections, Section B.1.a.).

   b. Selection Guidelines by Format or Type of Material:
   (See Rare Book Collections, Section IV.B.1.b.)

3. Reference/History of Medicine Collection:
   a. Categories:
   All substantive works relating to health and medicine from a historical perspective will be actively acquired. Although the primary language of these works will be English, representative or unique items will be collected in all languages. Other items of particular emphasis include:

   1) All reference works pertaining to the history of medicine and allied sciences, including bibliographic, biographical dictionaries, directories, and encyclopedias.

2) Journals in the history of medicine and allied sciences.

3) Publications on the history of books, printing, and illustration.

   b. Selection Guidelines by Format or Type of Material:
   (See Rare Book Collections, Section IV.B.1.b.)

4. Manuscripts and Archives Collection:
   a. Categories:
   Manuscripts and manuscript collections relating to American medicine from the seventeenth-century to present, with particular emphasis on Pennsylvania and Philadelphia, are actively acquired. European manuscripts are collected only in those areas relating to collection strength. The Library is particularly interested in acquiring the following:

   1) Student lecture notes (emphasis on 18th and 19th-century);

   2) Account books and daily journals;

   3) Diaries;

    4) Recipe books and formularies;

   5) Correspondence; and

   6) Collections of personal and professional papers.

The Historical Services Division of the Library houses the archives of the College of Physicians of Philadelphia. Archival material relating to the College that is actively collected includes:

   1) Correspondence or documentation relating to the operations of the College of Physicians;

   2) Minutes of meetings of College departments, divisions, sections, and committees;

   3) Printed programs of meetings and conferences sponsored by the College;

   4) College publications;

   5) Photographs and prints relating to the operations of the College;

   6) Cassette tapes and audiovisual tapes relating to the operation of the College; and

7) Ephemera commemorating or celebrating an event in the history of the College.

The archives of local medical societies and organizations, extinct and extant, are actively acquired. The records of national societies and organizations, extinct and extant, are acquired on a selective basis.

  b. Selection Guidelines by Format or Type of Material:
     (See Rare Book Collections, Section IV.B.1.b.)

 5. Photographs and Print Collection:
   a. Categories:
     Photographs and prints relating to the history of medicine are actively acquired. Emphasis is on American medicine, particularly as it relates to Philadelphia. Medical bookplates and public health posters are actively sought.

   b. Selection Guidelines by Format or Type of Material:
     (See Rare Book Collections, Section IV.B.1.b.)

 6. Special Collections:
   a. Categories:
     Within the Historical Services Division are a number of Special Collections including: William H. Helfand/Samuel X. Radbill Collection (medical bookplates); Samuel Lewis Collection (curios); Joseph Carson Collection (general medical history); Medical Autograph, William Kent Gilbert, and Hyde Collections (autographs of famous physicians); William N. Bradley Collection (portraits of famous physicians); Philadelphia General Hospital Collection (photograph archives); Samuel B. Sturgis Collection (prints and photographs of medical history); Faber Family Collection (medical illustrations); Samuel D. Gross Library (surgery); and Joseph T. Freeman Collection (gerontology).

   b. Selection Guidelines by Format or Type of Material:
     (See Rare Book Collections, Section IV.B.1.b.)

HOUSTON ACADEMY OF MEDICINE - TEXAS MEDICAL CENTER
(HOUSTON, TX)
LIBRARY

V. SPECIAL COLLECTIONS:
 A. Historical Research Center
  1. Rare Books
     The John P. McGovern History of Medicine Collection — this collection was originally formed when the Special Collections Department began in 1977 and the rare books from many divergent sources were brought together and made accessible for the clients. The collection was named for

Dr. McGovern in 1981 to honor his many years of financial support for the rare book collections and to recognize his gift of 650 titles from his personal collection. Today, the collection includes monographs, a few serial titles, some catalogs, selected encyclopedias, dictionaries, directories and a few secondary works in the history of medicine. The dates of publication of the titles range from the seventeenth century to the early twentieth century with the majority being published in the 19th century.

The major portion of the collection documents the growth and development of the medical specialties in the United States. The titles are in English and from American medical publishers. Titles from the publisher, Samuel Wood (later called Samuel and William Wood and then William Wood and Company), are of particular interest. The collection's strength is nineteenth-and early twentieth-century (Pre-WWI) holdings. Titles are actively sought for this portion of the McGovern Collection. The goal is to make this a research-level collection for our clients and a regional resource for the history of American medicine.

Cardiovascular medicine and surgery are two areas of special interest for the McGovern Collection. Because of the strong research, teaching, and patient care programs in the Texas Medical Center, acquisitions are not limited to the English language or to American publishers. Translations of classic texts, documentation on important firsts in these specialties, and secondary historical works are actively sought. The goal is to enhance and maintain this collection at the instructional support level.

Another portion of the McGovern Collection consists of medical classics and notable firsts in biomedical research and clinical care. This portion of the collection includes some reprints, such as the Sydenham Society publications, a few anatomical works, and other titles which are felt by the Director of the Historical Research Center to be of potential use for our clients' historical research. Titles from this part of the collection may be in English, French, German, or Latin and are acquired very selectively. Other smaller portions of the McGovern Collection include French medical texts (ca. 320 titles), the major portion of which were published between 1750 and 1850, a small selection (ca. 50 titles) in hematology, and some publications documenting early Texas medicine. Titles for this part of the collection are acquired very selectively. Preference is given to Texas medical serials and titles by French authors which are already in the collection.

The Burbank/Fraser Collection on Arthritis, Rheumatism and Gout— this collection is one of the finest in the world. The dates of publication in this collection range from sixteenth-century manuscripts to the mid-1950's with over fifteen languages represented in the texts. Monographs, offprints, reprints, serials, commercial catalogs, pamphlets, and other printed materials present researchers with information on rheumatic diseases from Hippocrates to Philip Hench. Information on all the rheumatic diseases is included; however, the collection is not as strong in scleroderma and the collagen diseases as the Gerald Rodnan Collection in Pittsburgh, Pennsylvania.

The major parts of this collection were acquired from Dr. Reginald Burbank (by purchase in 1952), from Dr. Kevin J. Fraser (by purchase in 1983), and from Dr. P. Kahler Hench (by gift in 1988). Materials in all languages, published or printed prior to 1958 are actively sought for this collection. The goal is to make the collection a comprehensive, national resource for research on the history of rheumatology and the rheumatic diseases.

The Mading Collection on Public Health—this collection documents early American public health conditions and infectious diseases. The collection was purchased for the Library in 1956 by the Cora and Webb Mading Foundation and is limited to United States imprints before 1926. The emphasis is on epidemiology, infectious diseases (excluding venereal diseases), sanitation, climatology as related to health, and government reports on health, mortality, and sanitation activities.

The majority of the collection is monographs, pamphlets, and city or state government reports which were published between 1770 and 1900. There is very little in the collection related to public health and infectious diseases in Texas. Titles are acquired for this collection when materials can be found which will complement its holdings and meet the selection criteria.

a. Selection criteria—emphasis is on acquiring materials which fall within the subject and date guidelines for the Library's existing collections. Materials are sought which will enhance the research potential of the historical collections and are likely to be used by students and health professionals in the Texas Medical Center for presentations and papers on clinical topics. Every effort is made to minimize duplication of titles held within the Library and, to some extent, within the Texas Medical Center libraries. The quality of the materials is determined by the condition of the paper, binding, and illustrations, by the uniqueness of the information, and by the reputation of the authors, illustrators, or editors. The price of an item is only one of many factors considered when reviewing items for inclusion in the historical collections.

b. Acquisitions—monographs, serials, and other printed materials for these collections are acquired from antiquarian book dealers, by transfer from the Library's general collection, and by gift. Materials to be purchased are selected by the Director of the Historical Research Center. The orders for items are reviewed by the Director of Collection Development and are sent to the vendors by the Acquisitions staff. In nearly all cases the Library purchases titles only from established antiquarian book dealers. Purchases from an individual are made only if and after the provenance of the materials is verified. Titles purchased by the

Library are received by the Acquisitions staff. Any questions about the titles received and fulfillment of the order are answered in consultation with the Director of the Historical Research Center. All payments for materials are handled following the Library's usual procedures for payment of invoices.

Suggestions on titles (monographs or serials) to be transferred to the Historical Research Center may come from Library staff or clients. Decisions about transfers will be made jointly by the Director of Collection Development and the Director of the Historical Research Center.

Donations of monographs, reprints, pamphlets, and other printed documents are accepted if the materials meet the selection criteria and enhance the existing collections. Materials which do not fall within the scope of existing historical collections will not be accepted without the consultation of the Library's Director, the Director of Collection Development, and, if appropriate, the Library's Board of Directors.

2. Historical photographs and graphic works

Photographs—the local history photographs and slides document a unique portion of our medical history. The collection contains portraits, construction photographs, views of the Texas Medical Center, images of buildings, and a limited number of images of interiors of hospitals or clinics. Most of the portraits are of Houston physicians. There are few portraits of nurses, health care administrators, or allied health personnel. Images are actively sought to fill gaps in this collection. The goal is to make this a recognized, regional resource on the history of the Texas Medical Center and the history of medicine in Houston.

Medical World News Collection—this collection was a gift from the owners of this journal, HEI, Inc., before the publication was sold. This collection is the backfile of images used to produce the journal from 1967 to 1975. Most of the images are arranged by a number assigned as each story was written for the journal. There are also a large number of images arranged by name or subject. The collection should be weeded for duplicate images and for images which were rented for one-time use. Acquisitions are not sought for this collection, although at some time the current owners of the journal may decide to add images to this collection. With weeding and cataloging, this collection has the potential to be a national resource on the history of twentieth-century American medicine.

Postcards—this collection (ca. 1000 images) exists to document Texas hospitals, medical or nursing schools, physicians' houses, spas or health resorts, sanitariums, state institutions, and federal health care facilities in the state. Cards are actively sought which were reproduced between 1880 and 1950. Real photographs or printed cards are acquired. The newer "chrome" or slick colored cards from the 1960's-1980's are collected only for Houston institutions.

Graphic works—this collection contains numerous other photographs and two-dimensional art work which has been donated to the Library as part of a manuscript or institutional collection. Examples of these are photographs from members of the Atomic Bomb Casualty Commission and photographs from Dr. E. J. Brewer of rheumatologists from throughout the world. The Director of the Historical Research Center or the Archivist in charge of processing an archival collection will determine whether photographs, prints, or other images will remain with the papers or records or should be transferred to the graphic works collection for preservation.

a. Selection criteria—emphasis is on acquiring materials which fall within the subject guidelines for the local history and postcard collections. Materials are sought which provide information and evidence concerning Harris County, Texas health care personnel and institutions and which will enhance the research potential of the collections. Black and white photographs are the preferred medium, although graphic works in many formats are accepted. The quality of the materials is determined by the condition of the paper or base film, the condition of the image, the clarity of the image, the uniqueness of the information, and by the supporting documentation accompanying the images.

b. Acquisitions—photographs, prints, slides, and most other graphic works are acquired for the Library's Historical Research Center through the solicitation of gifts. Except for the postcard collection, there are no funds allotted for the development of these collections. The Director of the Historical Research Center solicits the gifts and selects which unsolicited gifts can be accepted. Occasionally, postcards which fit into the scope of our collection are purchased by mail from vendors or from dealers at the annual postcard show and sales. Purchases are made only if funds are available in one of the accounts used for the development of the historical collections.

3. Harris County Medical Archive:

Institutional collections—these document the growth and development of local hospitals, schools and other health care organizations. Emphasis is on acquiring serial publications, occasional reports, and ephemeral printed materials from the Library's Participating and Supporting Institutions. Catalogs, annual reports, financial records, planning documents, newsletters, program brochures, telephone directories, and invitations are included in each of these collections. Materials in these collections are generally not the official records of the institutions. Gifts of archival records, historical files and photographs are accepted if there are resources available for preservation. The goal is to form a comprehensive historical collection on each institution and to make this a recognized, regional resource for the history of the Texas Medical Center and the history of health care in Houston. Materials are actively sought and donations are encouraged.

Research collections—these contain materials in many formats on a specific subject or with a unifying theme. Two examples of such collections are the Polio Collection, given to the Library by Dr. Joseph Melnick, and the NASA Space Life Sciences Archive. Additional research collections are not actively sought. Acceptance of such materials depends upon their comprehensiveness, uniqueness, future research value, and the availability of sufficient resources to preserve them properly and make them available for research.

Manuscript collections—these document the lives and careers of physicians and health care professionals in Harris County, Texas, of rheumatologists from throughout North America, and of members of the Atomic Bomb Casualty Commission. Correspondence, minutes of meetings, printed programs, unpublished papers, selected reprints, photographs, and other documents are found in most of the collections. These materials document the individuals' contributions to medicine or health care, their organizational affiliations, their families, and occasionally their philosophy. Additional collections are actively sought to enhance the depth of the coverage for Harris County and the comprehensiveness of the Library's coverage for rheumatology. The goal is to make these collections a recognized regional resource for Texas health care and a recognized national resource for rheumatology and the history of the rheumatic diseases.

a. Selection criteria—emphasis is on acquiring materials which fall within the guidelines for the Archive's institutional and manuscript collections. Materials which provide information and evidence about the Harris County health care community are actively sought. Reasonable efforts are made to minimize duplication of materials within the Archive and within the Library. The quality of the materials is determined by the uniqueness of the documentation, the condition of the materials, any restrictions on access and the provenance. Selection is not based upon the format of the materials. Many formats are acquired, with preference given to those whose documentation can be accessed directly by the researcher (e.g. printed documents are preferred over computer tapes). Research collections, except for additions to existing collections, are accepted only after careful consultation with the Library's Director, the Director of Collection Development and, if appropriate, the Library's Board of Directors. Whether any materials are accepted by the Library depends upon the availability of the resources to preserve the materials, upon the Library's ability to make them accessible for research, and upon a reasonable expectation that future resources will be available to maintain the materials.

b. Acquisitions—documents are acquired for the Harris County Medical Archive by gifts from institutions or from individuals. The solicitation, selection, and acceptance of the gifts is the responsibility of the Director of the Historical Research Center. No Library funds are used to purchase materials for the archive. The Library may, at the discretion of the Director of the Historical Research Center, decide to reimburse the donor for postage or shipping charges. Donors are encouraged not to restrict access to their materials for a long period of time; however, collections are accepted with reasonable restrictions which can be lifted after a period of time (usually 7-10 years).

Bibliography

This bibliography includes works which discuss general and theoretical aspects of collection development. Also included are works on these topics in health sciences libraries. More directed bibliographies appear at the end of each chapter. Those references, for the most part, are not repeated here.

Association of Research Libraries, Office of Management Studies, SPEC Kits. This series compiles from many U.S. academic libraries copies of procedures and policy statements on specific topics. Included in many of them are documents relating to or produced by health sciences libraries. Of particular relevance to collection development are the following titles:
    no. 11 Collection Development (1974)
    no. 38 Collection Development Policies (1977)
    no. 41 Collection Assessment (1978)
    no. 83 Approval Plans (1982)
    no. 111 Cooperative Collection Development (1985)
    no. 117 The Gifts & Exchange Function (1985)
    no. 131 Collection Development Organization and Staffing (1987)
    no. 137 Preservation Guidelines (1987)
    no. 141 Approval Plans (1988)
    no. 147 Serials Control and Deselection Projects (1988)
    no. 151 Qualitative Collection Analysis: The Conspectus Methodology (1989)
    no. 152 Brittle Books Programs (1989)
    no. 160 Preservation Organization and Staffing (1990)
    no. 162 Audiovisual Policies (1990)
    no. 169 Management of CD-ROM Databases (1990)
    no. 181 Performance Appraisal of Collection Development Librarians (1992)
    no. 195 Cooperative Strategies in Foreign Acquisitions (1993)
    no. 198 Automating Preservation Management (1993)
    no. 199 Video Collections and Multimedia (1993)
    no. 207 Organization of Collection Development (1995)
Atkinson RW. Old forms, new forms: the challenge of collection development. Coll Res Libr 1989 Sep;50(5):507-20.
Atkinson R. Text mutability and collection administration. Libr Acq Pract Theory 1990;14(4):355-8

American Library Association. Reference and Adult Services Division. Collection Development Policies Committee. The relevance of collection development policies: definition, necessity, and applications. RQ 1993 Fall;33(1):65-74.

Besson A, ed. Thornton's medical books, libraries and collectors: a study of bibliography and the book trade in relation to the medical sciences. 3rd. rev. ed. Brookfield, VT: Gower, 1990.

Bosch S, Promis P, Sugnet C. Guide to selecting and acquiring CD-ROMS, software, and other electronic publications. Chicago: American Library Association, 1994. (Acquisitions guidelines no. 9).

Brattan, Barry, et al. Selection and acquisition of AV material by health professionals, Bull Med Libr Assoc 1987 Oct;75(4):355-61.

Bryant B. ed. Guide for written collection policy statements. Chicago: American Library Association, 1989. (Collection management and development guides, no. 3)

Buckland MK. The roles of collections and the scope of collection development. J Docum 1989; 45(3):213-26.

Budd JM. Allocation formulas in the literature: a review. Libr Acq Pract Theory 1991;15(1):95-107.

Byrnes M, ed. Symposium: Preservation of the biomedical literature. Bull Med Libr Assoc 1989 Jul;77(3):256-298.

Chen CC. Biomedical, scientific, and technical book reviewing. Metuchen, NJ: Scarecrow Press, 1976.

Clark L, ed. Guide to review of library collections: preservation, storage, and withdrawal. Chicago: American Library Association, 1991. (Collection management and development guides, no. 5)

Colaianni LA. Peer review in journals indexed in Index Medicus. JAMA 1994 Jul 13; 72(2):156-8.

Corsi P, Weindling P, eds. Information sources in the history of medicine and science. London: Butterworth, 1983.

Craig DF, Strain PM. Analysis of collection development at the National Library of Medicine. Bull Med Libr Assoc 1980 Apr;68(2):197-206.

Demas S. Collection development for the electronic library: a conceptual and organizational model. Libr Hi Tech 1994;12(3):71-80.

Dombrowski T. Journal evaluation using journal citation reports as a collection development tool. Collection Manage 1988;10(3/4):175-80.

Eakin D. Health science library materials: collection development. In: Darling L, Bishop D, Colaianni, LA, eds. Handbook of medical library practice. 4th ed. v.2. Chicago: Medical Library Association, 1983:27-91.

Evans RW. Collection development policy statements: the documentation process. Collection Manage 1985; 7(1):63-73.

Evans GE. Developing library and information center collections. 2nd ed. Littleton, CO: Libraries Unlimited, 1987.

Faigel M. Methods and issues in collection evaluation today. Libr Acq Pract Theory 1985; 9(1):21- 35.

Ferguson AW. Assessing the collection development need for CD-ROM products. Libr Acq Pract Theory 1988; 12(3/4):325-32.

Futas E, Intner S, eds. Collection evaluation. Libr Trends 1985 Winter; 33(3):237-436.

Gorman GE, Howes BR. Collection development for libraries. London: Bowker-Saur, 1989.

Gorman PN, Ash J, Wykoff L. Can primary care physicians' questions be answered using the medical literature? Bull Med Libr Assoc 1994 Apr;82(2):140-6.

Hall BH. Collection assessment manual for college and university libraries. Phoenix, AZ: Oryx Press, 1985.

Haselbauer KJ. A research guide to the health sciences: medical, nutritional, and environmental. New York: Greenwood Press, 1987. (Reference sources for the social sciences and humanities. no. 4.)

Hattendorf LC. The art of reference collection development. RQ 1989; 29(2):219-29.

Hazen D. Collection development policies in the information age. Coll Res Libr 1995 Jan;56(1):31- 7.

Henderson A. Forecasting changes in periodical prices. Ser Libr 1992; 21(4):33-43.

Higginbotham BB, Bowdoin S. Access versus assets: a comprehensive guide to resource sharing for academic librarians. Chicago: American Library Association, 1993. (Frontiers of access to library materials, no. 1)

Hoolihan C. Collection development policies in medical rare book collections. Collection Manage 1989;11(3/4):167-79.

Jenkins C, Morley M, eds. Collection management in academic libraries. Aldershot, England: Gower, 1991.

Johnson P, Intner SS. Recruiting, education, and training librarians for collection development. Westport, CT: Greenwood Press, 1994.

Kaag CS, Cann SL, eds. Collection evaluation techniques: a short selective, practical current annotated bibliography, 1980-90. Chicago: Reference and Adult Services Division, American Library Association, 1991. (RASD occasional papers, no. 10)

Kernaghan SG, Giloth BE. Consumer health information: managing hospital-based centers. Chicago: Hospital Research and Educational Trust, American Hospital Association, 1992.

King DW, McDonald DD, Roderer NK. Scientific journals in the United States: their production, use and economics. Stroudsburg, PA: Hutchinson Ross, 1981.

Kronick DA. A history of scientific and technical periodicals: the origins and development of the scientific and technical press, 1665-1790. 2nd ed. Metuchen, NJ: Scarecrow Press, 1976.

Kronick DA. The literature of the life sciences. Philadelphia: ISI Press, 1985.

Lancaster FW. If you want to evaluate your library... 2nd ed. Champaign: Univ. of Illinois, Graduate School of Library and Information Science, 1993.

Lockett B, ed. Guide to the evaluation of library collections. Chicago: American Library Association, 1989. (Collection management and development guides, no. 2)

Losee RM. Theoretical adequacy and the scientific study of materials selection. Collection Manage 1988;10(3/4):15-26.

Magrill RM, Hickey DJ. Acquisitions management and collection development in libraries. 2nd ed. Chicago: American Library Association, 1989.

Marshall JG. The impact of the hospital library on clinical decision making: the Rochester study. Bull Med Libr Assoc 1992 Apr;80(2):169-78.

McClung PA, ed. Selection of library materials in the humanities, social sciences, and sciences. Chicago: American Library Association, 1985.

Meadows AJ. Development of science publishing in Europe. Amsterdam: Elsevier, 1980.

Morton LT, Godbolt S, eds. Information sources in the medical sciences. 4th ed. London: Bowker-Saur, 1992.

Morse DH, Richards DT. Collection development policies for health sciences libraries. Chicago: Medical Library Association, 1992. (MLA DocKit, no. 3)

Mosher PH. Quality and library collections: new directions in research and practice in collection evaluation. Adv Libr 1984; 13:211-38.

Mosher PH, Pankake M. A guide to coordinated and cooperative collection development. Libr Res Tech Serv 1983 Oct;27(4):417-31.

Nisonger TE. Collection evaluation in academic libraries: a literature guide and annotated bibliography. Englewood, CO: Libraries Unlimited, 1992.

Norman JM, ed. Morton's medical bibliography: an annotated checklist of texts illustrating the history of medicine (Garrison and Morton) 5th ed. London: Scolar Press, 1991.

Osburn CB, Atkinson RW. Collection management: a new treatise. Greenwich CT: JAI Press, 1991. (Foundations in library information science, v. 26A-B)

Overmier J, Mueller MH. Collection development policies and practices in medical school rare book libraries. Bull Med Libr Assoc 1984 Apr;72(2):150-54.

Pankake M. From book selection to collection management: continuity and advance in an unending work. Adv Libr 1984; 13:185-210.

Powell N, ed. Pacific Northwest collection assessment manual. 3rd ed. Salem: Oregon State Library Foundation, 1990.

Rees A, ed. The consumer health information source book. 4th ed. Phoenix, AZ: Oryx Press, 1994.

Richards, DT. Collection development in health sciences libraries: a report on the Medical Library Association post conference, May 31-June 1, 1985, New York City. Libr Acq Pract Theory 1985; 9(4):351-4. (A brief summary of the only conference devoted to collection development in health sciences libraries. The full proceedings of the conference were published as an audiotape set from MLA.)

Riley RA, Shipman BL. Building and maintaining a library gopher - traditional skills applied to emerging resources. Bull Med Assoc 1995 Apr; 83(2):221-7.

Roper FW, Boorkman JA. Introduction to reference sources in the health sciences. 3rd ed. Metuchen, NJ: Medical Library Association and Scarecrow Press, 1994.

Rutledge J, Swindler L. The selection decision: defining criteria and establishing priorities. Coll Res Libr 1987 Mar;48(2):123-31.

Sanders NP, O'Neill ET, Weibel ST. Automated collection analysis using the OCLC and RLG bibliographic databases. Coll Res Libr 1988 Jul;49(4):305-14.

Schaffner AC. The future of scientific journals: lessons from the past. Info Tech Libr 1994 Dec;13(4):239-47.

Schwartz CA. Book selection, collection development, and bounded rationality. Coll Res Libr 1989 May;50(3):328-43.

Sellen BC, Curly A. The collection building reader. New York: Neal-Schuman, 1992.

Shreeves E, ed. Guide to budget allocation for information resources. Chicago: American Library Association, 1991. (Collection management and development guides, no. 4)

Spiller D. Book selection: an introduction to principles and practice. 4th ed. London: Clive Bingley, 1986.

Stebelman S. The role of subject specialists in reference collection development. RQ 1989 Winter; 29(2):266-73.

Steuart RD, Miller GB. Collection development in libraries: a treatise. Greenwich, CT: JAI Press, 1980. (Foundations in library and information science, v. 10A-B)

Tenopir C. Online databases: collection development. Libr J 1990 Sep 1; 115(14):194-97.

Van Orden P, Phillips EB, eds. Background readings in building library collections. New York: Scarecrow, 1979.

Walker RD, Hunt CD. Scientific and technical literature: an introduction to forms of communication. Chicago: American Library Association, 1990.

Walter PL. Doing the unthinkable: canceling journals in a research library. Serials Libr 1990;18(1/2):141-53.

Warren KS. Coping with the biomedical literature: a primer for the scientist and the clinician. New York: Praeger, 1981.

Welsch EK. Back to the future: a personal statement on collection development in an information culture. Libr Res Tech Serv 1989 Jan;33(1):29-36.

Wortman WA. Collection management: background and principles. Chicago: American Library Association, 1989.

Zinn NW. Special collections: history of health science collections, oral history, archives and manuscripts. In: Darling L, Bishop D, Colaianni LA, eds. Handbook of medical library practice. 4th ed. v. 3. Chicago: Medical library Association, 1988:469-572.

Glossary

AAAS	American Association for the Advancement of Science
AAMC	Association of American Medical Colleges
AAP	Association of American Publishers
ACS	American Chemical Society
ALA	American Library Association
ALCTS	Association for Library Collections and Technical Services (ALA)
ARL	Association of Research Libraries
AVLINE	Audiovisuals Online (database—NLM)
BIOSIS	BioSciences Information Services
BRS	Bibliographic Retrieval Services (online service now called CDP Online)
CAP	Cooperative Acquisitions Program
CATLINE	Cataloging Online (database—NLM)
CD-ROM	Compact Disc, Read-Only Memory
CE	Continuing education
CINAHL	Cumulative Index to Nursing and Allied Health Literature
CONTU	Commission on New Technological Uses of Copyrighted Works
COSAP	Cooperative Serials Acquisitions Program
E.T. Net	Educational Technology Network (NLM)
FAX	Telefacsimile
GenBank	Genetic Sequences Data Bank
GUI	Graphical User Interface
HSN	Hospital Satellite Network
IEEE	Institute of Electrical and Electronics Engineers
ILL	Interlibrary loan

Internet	Network of networks using standard telecommunications protocol
ISI	Institute for Scientific Information
JCAHO	Joint Commission on Accreditation of Healthcare Organizations
LC	Library of Congress
MEDLINE	MEDLARS Online (database—NLM)
MeSH	Medical Subject Headings (NLM)
MLA	Medical Library Association
MLCNY	Medical Library Center of New York
NAL	National Agricultural Library
NASA	National Aeronautics and Space Administration
NASIG	North American Serials Interest Group
NIH	National Institutes of Health
NLM	National Library of Medicine
OCLC	Online Computer Library Center
PCR	Primary Collection Responsibility (RLG)
PDR	Physicians Desk Reference
PSRMLS	Pacific Southwest Regional Medical Library Service
PsycINFO	Psychological Information (database—American Psychological Association)
RECBIR	Regional Coordination of Biomedical Information Resources
RIME	Research in Medical Education (AAMC)
RLG	Research Libraries Group
RML	Regional Medical Library
SCAMC	Symposium on Computer Applications in Medical Care
SERHOLD	Serials Holdings Online (database—NLM)
SERLINE	Serials Online (database—NLM)
UC	University of California
VHS	Video Home System

Index

This is primarily a subject index. Personal authors of references cited in the text are not indexed. Acronyms and initialisms are given preference as indexing terms if more commonly used than full names of organizations or publications.

Author Biographies

Dottie Eakin is Director of the Medical Sciences Library, Texas A&M University. Previously she has held positions in library administration and collection development at the University of Michigan and the Houston Academy of Medicine-Texas Medical Center Library. She authored the chapter on collection development in the 4th edition of the *Handbook of Medical Library Practice,* and with Pat Walter developed the MLA CE course on Writing for Publication: the professional article. She is the 1991 recipient of the Louise Darling Medal for Distinguished Achievement in Collection Development in the Health Sciences.

Daniel T. Richards served as Director of Biomedical Libraries at Dartmouth from 1991-1995. Previous positions included Collection Development Officer at the National Library of Medicine (NLM) from 1988-91, Assistant Health Sciences Librarian at Columbia University from 1981-1988, and a variety of positions over a ten-year period at the UCLA Louise Darling Biomedical Library. He served as a guest lecturer in the library schools at UCLA, Columbia University, and Catholic University, and was a continuing education instructor for the Medical Library Association (MLA). An active member of MLA and ALA, Richards served on several national committees, including a three year term on MLA's Board of Directors. He presented papers at national and international conferences, and has been a consultant to booksellers, universities and publishers. He was the author of more than forty articles, book chapters, and reports, and with David Morse compiled *Collection Development Policies in Health Sciences Libraries,* published by MLA in 1992. Richards was chosen as an NLM Associate in 1970-71, and was awarded MLA's Louise Darling Medal for Distinguished Achievement in Collection Development in the Health Sciences in 1989.